Praise for *The Mission Is Remission*...

"Pat Williams' new book will be extremely valuable to families dealing with a cancer situation. I have learned that early detection and powerful prayer warriors are two key elements in my cancer battle. Pat covers these two topics and many more."

Digger Phelps
Former Notre Dame Head Basketball Coach
ESPN College Basketball Analyst

"Pat Williams, a man of great strength and faith, has written an enormously useful book for people who have contracted cancer. Be it the importance of optimism, the value of family, the significance of faith—whatever one's faith may be—or the curative power of friendship, the advice Pat offers are universal gifts to all of us living with cancer. I wish I had this book to read when I contracted multiple myeloma seven years ago."

Tom Meschery, NBA 1961-1971
Author of *Nothing You Lose Can Be Replaced* and *Some Men*

"As a fellow cancer survivor, I have a great heart for Pat Williams' story. This book will inspire families everywhere to keep battling and never give up the fight."

Eric Davis
Former Major League Baseball All-Star

"This book is awesome. My wife and I couldn't put it down. It's well-written and packed with so much good information for anyone dealing with a cancer battle."

Mel Stottlemyre
Former New York Yankees Pitcher

"Having a positive attitude and a valuable mission in life is half the battle in beating cancer. When it comes to living a hopeful, meaningful life on a daily basis, Pat Williams is a shining example. Despite battling a disease that has scientists and clinicians working around the clock to beat, he has the unique ability of always seeing the glass as being half full. Pat continues to be an inspiration to thousands touched by fatal cancers like multiple myeloma."

Kathy Giusti
Founder and CEO, MMRF and MMRC

"Pat Williams' book is filled with encouragement, insight and realistic hope. If you are battling cancer, or know someone who is, this book is a must-read."

Senator Bob Dole

"My wife and I have read *The Mission Is Remission* and both of us loved it. This is a book that will offer a lot of hope and practical help to those battling cancer and other challenges in life."

Chuck Pagano
Indianapolis Colts Head Coach

"I have experienced thousands of battles on the ice during my hockey career, but none compared with my battle with cancer. Read Pat Williams' account with his struggle with multiple myeloma. It's a positive story and will give you great hope with your life challenges."

Mario Lemieux
Hockey Hall-of-Famer
Pittsburgh Penguins Owner

"I believe we go through what we go through to help others get through what we went through. In *The Mission Is Remission*, Pat Williams shares what he has gone through in his cancer battle to help you fight your cancer battle. This book is a difference-maker!"

Jay Carty
Former Los Angeles Laker

"Pat's six factors will help you maximize your quality of life for the maximum time. And, when it comes right down to it, that's all any of us are striving to do in life—whether we're trying to put the full-court press on cancer or rising to the challenge of change. This book is all about how to win, regardless of your prognosis."

Alan Hobson
Two-Time Cancer Survivor and
Climb Back from Cancer Coach
Author, *Climb Back from Cancer*

"This insightful book by Pat Williams hit the nail on the head as it relates to the reality of suffering from any form of cancer. It should serve as encouragement to those who are fighting the battle and it certainly puts things in perspective regarding life's priorities. Thanks, Pat, for sharing."

Jerry Colangelo
Director of USA Basketball

"I know from personal experience that when you are told you have cancer, you immediately feel so alone. Pat Williams' comforting words puncture that wall with his customary grace, empowering us to live with the courage he personifies daily."

Ed Randall
"Ed Randall's Talking Baseball" on WFAN-Radio

"The fear of hearing the diagnosis of cancer, the glee in knowing you've won the initial battle with this terrible disease and the faith required to manage both is something I'm very familiar with. I admire Pat for his tireless efforts in support of both cancer survivors and those searching for a cure. I'm sure that after reading this book you will share my admiration and Pat's passion."

Jerry Dipoto
General Manager, Los Angeles Angels of Anaheim

"As he does so frequently Pat eloquently lays out the range of emotions that have been real to all of us who have heard the 'C' word. Once hearing that word, Pat does what makes him special—he stays positive and projects that attitude in a way that impacts all! This book is the beautiful extension of that. What a compelling read filled with optimism."

Don Yaeger
New York Times bestselling author

"When I received my cancer diagnosis years ago, it was a life-changing experience for me. I realized, for the first time, that I am not invincible and I learned to appreciate life a whole lot more after I realized I could be taken quickly. Pat Williams has captured those thoughts in his new book, *The Mission Is Remission*. It is highly recommended reading for all of us, cancer patients or not."

John Kruk
ESPN Baseball Analyst

"In order to overcome a cancer diagnosis, one has to have faith, a selfless caregiver and a plan. *The Mission Is Remission* helps you focus on developing *your* individual plan for combating cancer. Pat Williams is a parent, an educator, a cancer survivor and one of the world's most admired figures for helping others. He has once again found a way to help others with *The Mission Is Remission*."

Harry Rhoads, Jr.
CEO of Washington Speakers Bureau
and four-time cancer survivor

THE MISSION IS REMISSION

HOPE FOR BATTLING CANCER

Pat Willium
2014

PAT WILLIAMS

with **JIM DENNEY**

Foreword by **ARNOLD PALMER**

Health Communications, Inc.
Deerfield Beach, Florida

www.hcibooks.com

**Library of Congress Cataloging-in-Publication Data
is available through the Library of Congress**

© 2014 Pat Williams

ISBN-13: 9780757317828 (Paperback)
ISBN-10: 0757317820 (Paperback)
ISBN-13: 9780757317835 (ePub)
ISBN-10: 0757317839 (ePub)

Publisher: Health Communications, Inc.
      3201 S.W. 15th Street
      Deerfield Beach, FL 33442–8190

Cover image ©Vladimir Rojas
Cover design by Dane Wesolko
Interior design and formatting by Lawna Patterson Oldfield

To Dr. Robert Reynolds and Dr. Yasser Khaled,
the two oncologists who have treated me for the past
three years. I'm grateful for their skill, their compassion,
their insight, and the gift of life and hope they
have given me. This book is also dedicated to the nurses
who went far beyond the call of duty to provide
care and encouragement to me through the
most difficult crisis of my life.

CONTENTS

ACKNOWLEDGMENTS

With deep appreciation, I acknowledge the support and guidance of the following people who helped make this book possible:

Special thanks to Alex Martins, Dan DeVos, and Rich DeVos of the Orlando Magic.

Hats off to my assistant, Andrew Herdliska; my proofreader, Ken Hussar; and my ace typist, Fran Thomas. Thanks also to my writing partner, Jim Denney, for his superb contributions in shaping this manuscript.

Hearty thanks also go to Peter Vegso and his outstanding team at HCI for their vision and insight, and for believing that we had something important to say in these pages.

A special measure of gratitude goes to those who agreed to be interviewed for this book, and who generously shared their experience and insights: Kathy Giusti, Andrew Herdliska,

Audra Hollifield, Pastor Randall James, Dr. Robert Reynolds, my daughter Karyn, and my sister Ruthie.

And, finally, special thanks and appreciation go to my wife, Ruth, and to my wonderful and supportive family. The joy they bring me makes life worth living—and worth fighting for.

FOREWORD

We have to stick together.

We who are battling cancer, we cancer survivors, we who are caring for friends or family members with cancer—we all have to stick together. We need to share our strength and hope with each other. And that's what Pat Williams has done in his book *The Mission Is Remission.*

I have a grudge against cancer. I hate it with a passion. Cancer has hit me, my family, and many close friends. I lost my first wife to cancer.

No one is safe from this disease, no matter how young we are, no matter how much we exercise and avoid smoking and other carcinogens. Cancer can strike anyone.

I have a daughter who was diagnosed with breast cancer when she was just thirty-two—and she's a cancer survivor today. I was in my late sixties when I had surgery for prostate cancer at the Mayo Clinic—yet the patient in the room next to mine was having the same surgery, and he was a minister, just twenty-nine years old.

So no one is immune. We all need to be on our guard against this disease. We have to get regular physicals and tests so that if cancer strikes, we can detect it early. If we are diagnosed with cancer, we have to face it realistically, with hope and optimism. We have to fight back with all our might.

> If we are diagnosed with cancer, we have to face it realistically, with hope and optimism. We have to fight back with all our might.

That's why this book, *The Mission Is Remission*, is so important. Pat Williams has generously opened up his life and taken us inside his cancer battle. In this book, he shows us how to face cancer with courage and a can-do attitude. He also shows us how to get the most out of life, even while battling cancer.

Whether you are a cancer patient, a cancer survivor, or a friend to someone who's been diagnosed with this disease, you need this book. These pages are brimming with optimism and hope. In fact, this may be the most positive and inspiring book ever written on the subject of cancer. It will make you laugh, it will make you strong, it will encourage you.

Pat's message is just what the doctor ordered.

To your good health!

—**Arnold Palmer**
March 2014

INTRODUCTION:
A SHATTERING DIAGNOSIS

My world changed on January 7, 2011.

I spent the entire day, from 7:00 AM to 5:00 PM, under-going an intensive physical assessment at Florida Hospital's Celebration Health Assessment Center. It was extremely thorough—the kind of going-over you'd receive at the Mayo Clinic. The Orlando Magic's human resources director, Audra Hollifield, had arranged for all the executives of the Magic organization to undergo this assessment. Though I was there for a complete physical, not for any specific problem or complaint, I hoped that the doctors at Celebration would uncover the reason for the nagging back pain that had plagued me for weeks.

After I'd been thoroughly poked, prodded, monitored, and sampled, Dr. Christine Edwards told me, "Pat, it all looks good—except there's something in your blood work we're not sure about. You should get that checked by your primary physician."

Something in your blood work we're not sure about. Those words didn't seem ominous at the time, and I hardly gave them any thought. I didn't know it then, but those words were about to completely upend my world.

Except for that seemingly insignificant detail in my blood work, I received a clean bill of health. Two days later, on Sunday, January 9, 2011, I ran in the eighteenth running of the Walt Disney World Marathon—my fifty-eighth marathon. At age seventy, I had been running marathons for fifteen years, and this was one of my best marathons ever. I felt good throughout the race. Sure, I had the usual soreness in my limbs afterward, but nothing out of the ordinary.

Three days after the marathon, I woke up with crippling pain radiating from my spine. I was in agony. I couldn't get out of bed, couldn't even move. I had never felt such pain, even after a marathon. I suspected a herniated disk, a pulled muscle, or a nerve problem, and I immediately made an appointment with a back specialist. After extensive x-rays and an MRI, the doctors said they could find no problem with my back.

On Thursday, January 13, I went to see my primary care physician, Dr. Vince Wilson. By that time, he had received the report on the blood work from my physical at Celebration.

Dr. Wilson sat me down. His expression was troubled. He said, "Why do bad things happen to all the good people?"

Dr. Wilson sat me down. His expression was troubled. He said, "Why do bad things happen to all the good people?"

"What do you mean, Doc?"

"There's something in your blood work, Pat—an abnormal kind of protein called a paraprotein. I have a strong suspicion, though I hope I'm wrong. I'm going to refer you to a leading expert in this field, Dr. Robert Reynolds."

Dr. Wilson made an appointment for me with Dr. Reynolds for the next Monday, January 17. Over the weekend, I began preparing myself mentally and emotionally for bad news.

Before my appointment with Dr. Reynolds, I wasn't even sure what his field of medical specialization was. Arriving at his office, I saw that he was an oncologist and hematologist— a specialist in cancer and diseases of the blood. When I met him, he told me he'd been an Orlando Magic fan and season-ticket holder for years. He knew who I was and he remembered those early days in the 1980s when I was working hard to bring an NBA franchise to Orlando.

At first, Dr. Reynolds thought I had come merely to rule out any serious illness. But after he saw my blood work, his tone became somber and he got right down to business.

"Pat," he said, "it looks like you have multiple myeloma—a cancer of the plasma cells in the blood and bone marrow."

When he said that, both my blood and my bone marrow turned to ice, even though I didn't know what multiple myeloma was. To be honest, I didn't want to know. Yes, Dr. Reynolds had called it "cancer." But I quickly put the "C word" out of my mind. I seized on Dr. Reynolds's phrase "it looks like," interpreting it as though he wasn't certain, the blood test might be wrong, and I might not have the C word after all.

"We'll do some tests right away," Dr. Reynolds continued, "and I'll let you know next week exactly what we're dealing with." The tests involved a full-body x-ray of my skeleton and an extraction of bone marrow from my hip.

The fact that Dr. Reynolds was still doing tests gave me hope—even a sense of denial—that his initial impression might be wrong. Maybe this wasn't multiple myeloma after all. A blood test didn't prove anything, right? I told myself that when the x-ray and bone marrow tests were completed, Dr. Reynolds would say something like, "Oops, that initial diagnosis was a mistake. Sorry I gave you a scare, Pat, but we needed to rule it out." I was sure it would turn out to be nothing at all.

I went home that evening and didn't say a word to my wife, Ruth, about what Dr. Reynolds had told me. I said to myself, *Why get Ruth worried and upset over a diagnosis that's going to turn out false anyway?* But as the day of my next appointment with Dr. Reynolds approached, the thought nagged at me, *What if it turns out to be true?* Just in case this thing turned out to be multiple whatchamacallit, maybe it would be a good idea to have Ruth at my side when the doctor gave me the news.

I asked Ruth to go with me to my next appointment. She seemed baffled by my request. I had never asked her to go with me to a doctor's appointment before, but she agreed to go. On the day of the appointment, we got into the car and started off for Dr. Reynolds's office. As we drove, Ruth said, "Now, where are we going?"

I handed her a letter I had received from Dr. Reynolds's office, confirming my appointment. She unfolded it and looked at the letterhead—Dr. Robert B. Reynolds, Oncology and Hematology.

"Pat," she said, a look of shock on her face, "he's an oncologist. This is cancer!"

"Oh, no," I said, "it's nothing like that. It's just something they found in my blood. Let's just go see what the doctor says. If there's a problem, we'll face it when the time comes."

A few minutes later, we arrived at Dr. Reynolds's office and sat down to discuss my case with the doctor.

"It's definite, Pat," Dr. Reynolds began, straight from the shoulder. "It's cancer. You have multiple myeloma."

*"When the radiologist told me
I had invasive cancer, I walked down
the hospital corridor. . . . I could almost
see the fear coming toward me
like a big, black shadow."*

—Geraldine Brooks

The Mission Is Remission

I was shell-shocked. Looking back, it seems ridiculous that I was so surprised. Dr. Reynolds had tried to prepare me. He had told me that the initial tests indicated multiple myeloma. Though I thought at the time that I was facing the diagnosis squarely, I realize now that there was a huge zone of denial in my thinking. I was protecting myself from the truth by telling myself the initial blood work was a mistake.

People tend to think that denial is a bad thing—and it can be, if taken to such an extreme that people simply refuse to face reality. But a certain amount of denial can be useful in protecting us and helping us to cope with bad news. Anyone facing cancer needs to have hope, and sometimes a spoonful of denial can go a long way toward maintaining a much-needed positive outlook.

At that moment, as I sat in Dr. Reynolds's office, hearing my diagnosis, I was suddenly robbed of all my denial. The facts were stark. I had cancer. It was the most devastating news I had ever received. Dr. Reynolds passed me the Kleenex box. I took a tissue, mopped my eyes, and began mentally planning my own funeral.

I don't think I realized at the time what an emotional shock it was for Ruth. Fortunately, her instinctive response to a crisis is to immediately try to understand the problem, gather all the facts, and find solutions. Ruth is a consultant with Franklin Covey and an expert on resource management who has consulted with Fortune 500 companies. I was glad to have her there, not only for emotional support, but for her keen problem-solving ability. Ruth took out her notepad and began asking questions and taking notes on everything the doctor said.

"Dr. Reynolds," Ruth said, "this doesn't even seem possible. Pat has taken better care of himself than any human being I know. He never puts anything bad into his system. And as for exercise, he runs marathons—he's a fitness nut! How could this happen? What caused it?"

"We don't know," Dr. Reynolds said. "Sometimes age is a factor, but we're discovering more and more that there are increasing numbers of young people being diagnosed with multiple myeloma. This is not a common disease in the population at large, but as a specialist in blood disorders,

I see myeloma on a fairly regular basis. Fortunately, there's been a lot of research on this disease over the past couple of decades. Because of that research and the new treatments that are available, we've been seeing myeloma patients living progressively longer. So there's a very good chance that you can live a long time, and you can live a fairly normal life."

"Doc," I said, "that's great to hear. I have a very active life as a sports executive, public speaker, and author, and I really want to be able to maintain that lifestyle. So what do I do now? How do we cure it?"

"Pat, I'm afraid multiple myeloma isn't curable—but it's very treatable. The goal of treatment is remission. With chemotherapy, you'll have a good chance of remission. And there are new therapies being developed all the time. You'd much rather have multiple myeloma today than twenty years ago—that's how far medical science has come."

Dr. Reynolds went on to explain the nature of multiple myeloma and the treatment plan he recommended. In the midst of my shock, I tried to process everything he told me. I asked questions and tried to focus on the answers.

Fortunately, Ruth was able to take it all in much better than I was. She asked insightful questions, and then took good notes on the answers. Her ability to sift the information, ask the right questions, and record Dr. Reynolds's answers was crucial. Over the days and weeks that followed, there were literally hundreds of times when I asked Ruth, "Now, tell me again, what did Dr. Reynolds say about such-and-such? What did he advise about so-and-so?" And Ruth had all the answers in her notes.

Dr. Reynolds took his time explaining everything we needed to know about multiple myeloma, and helped me to understand the course of treatment that lay ahead. Near the end of our conversation, he smiled reassuringly and added, "Pat, I honestly think you're going to do well with this."

"I will? Why do you think so?"

"From what I know about you by seeing you in the media, plus the short time we've talked together, I think you're going to handle this challenge well. I base that on six factors. First, your positive attitude is very important. Second, your good fitness level is an important factor—I don't get to treat many marathoners. Third, your strong faith is going to be a powerful factor. Fourth, the love of your family is a huge factor. Fifth, you have many caring friends, especially in the Magic organization. And sixth, the support of the Orlando community will be a very positive factor. The people of Central Florida are going to rally around you in a mighty way. With these six factors going for you, plus excellent medical care, I think you have a very good chance of remission."

> An inspiration struck me: "How about this for a motivational slogan, Doc: The Mission Is Remission?"

At that point, An inspiration struck me: "How about this for a motivational slogan, Doc: The Mission Is Remission?"

"I like it," he said.

"What's our next move, Doc?"

"We'll start chemotherapy and move as quickly and aggressively as we can."

"That's what I like to hear. Okay, Dr. Reynolds. I'm in your hands. I'll be an obedient patient. Let's get going."

An Unflinching Look at Cancer

I had never given much thought to cancer until I received this diagnosis. I wasn't aware of any family history of cancer. I've been a health, diet, and fitness fanatic all my life. I've never smoked or chewed tobacco, and I've never used alcohol. I've always exercised religiously. You can't run marathons at age seventy without being in better-than-average physical shape. I had none of the risk factors generally associated with cancer, so the possibility simply didn't cross my mind.

But the reality is that no one is immune from cancer. According to the National Cancer Institute, men have a 44.8 percent risk of developing some form of cancer in their lifetime (nearly a 1 in 2 chance) , and a 23.1 percent risk of dying from some form of cancer (about a 1 in 4 chance). And women have a 38.2 percent risk of developing cancer in their lifetime (more than a 1 in 3 chance), and a 19.4 percent risk of dying from cancer (a 1 in 5 chance).[1]

An unflinching look at those statistics will tell you that, at some point in your life, you will either be diagnosed with cancer yourself, or someone close to you will be. So I have written this book for three groups of people: (1) people with cancer, (2) people who love someone who has cancer, and (3) people who are healthy now but who know that cancer may play a role in their lives someday. In short, this book is for everyone. It doesn't matter whether you are young or old, male or female, tall or short, heavy or thin, smoker or nonsmoker, drinker or nondrinker, I have written this book with you in mind.

One way or another, cancer *will* be a factor in your life. But experience has shown that the more we understand about cancer, the less terror it holds. Cancer is a deadly disease, to be sure, but the statistics prove that nearly two-thirds of all cancer patients are still alive five years after their initial diagnosis. The treatments and survival rates are getting better all the time.[2]

---

*"Cancer is the ultimate nemesis
that hangs in the balance for one in
three women and one in two
men in their lifetime."*

—David Agus, M.D.

What is cancer? It's a broad class of diseases that involve the destructive and out-of-control growth of cells. Medical science refers to cancer as a "malignant neoplasm." "Malignant" means "causing harm or suffering," while "neoplasm" comes from the Greek and means "new or changed tissue." In most forms of cancer, cells begin to divide and grow uncontrollably, and these cells become malignant tumors that spread and invade other parts of the body, usually by moving through the lymphatic system or bloodstream. There are at least two hundred distinct forms of cancer that can occur in the human body.

The vast majority of cancers can be traced to environmental exposure (radiation, asbestos, and other pollutants), lifestyle factors (such as diet, smoking, drinking, and obesity), oncoviruses (cancer-causing viruses such as human papilloma virus), and so on. While the vast majority of cancers are due to our environment and the substances we ingest, a small minority of cancer deaths (5 to 10 percent) are traceable to inherited genetic defects.

Because I have always treated my body as a temple, I have often asked myself and my doctors, "Why did I get cancer? How did this happen?" Is my cancer the result of an inherited genetic defect? Maybe. My mother's mother died of cancer. According to the doctors at that time, it was a cancer in her colon that followed an unusual course by metastasizing into her bone marrow. But is that true? So little was known about cancer in those days that it's conceivable she had undiagnosed multiple myeloma. Did I inherit a genetic predisposition to this disease? The truth is that I will never know.

Then again, there might have been an environmental factor I'm not aware of. For example, I do a lot of flying. While I was on board an airliner cruising at 30,000 feet, a stray cosmic ray particle might have come in from outer space, flashed through my body at the speed of light, and damaged the genetic material in one cell of my bone marrow, causing a mutation that led to cancer. But once again, I'll never know.

The doctors can't explain why I have cancer, and ultimately, it doesn't matter why. Regardless of what kind of cancer a person has, the "why" question just doesn't matter. Nonsmokers sometimes get lung cancer. People who are extremely careful about their diet sometimes get digestive tract cancers. Men sometimes get breast cancer. And innocent little children get leukemia.

In July 2011, my friend Bob Hewitt, a former part-owner of the Orlando Magic, was diagnosed with lung cancer, even though he had never been a smoker. Two months after his diagnosis, Bob passed away. Sometimes cancer happens, and there simply is no "why" that makes any sense or offers any comfort. In fact, it's the seemingly random way cancer chooses its victims that makes this disease so frightening to most of us.

> For you and me as cancer patients, or as loved ones of cancer patients, it's not important how we got here. The only thing that matters is where we go from here.

We want to know why, but once the diagnosis has been confirmed, the "why" question serves no useful purpose for the individual who suffers from cancer. Yes, researchers need to ask the "why" question—and we pray that they find the ultimate answers so that all forms of cancer may finally be prevented and cured. But for you and me as cancer patients, or as loved ones of cancer patients, it's not important how we got here. The only thing that matters is where we go from here. And that's what this book is about.

The day Dr. Reynolds told me I had cancer, he also gave me hope. He said, "Pat, I honestly think you're going to do well with this." And he told me that he based that message of hope on six factors, which he listed for me. In the rest of this book, I am going to explore the six factors that gave me hope that I could be victorious in my battle against cancer. Each of the following chapters explores one of those six factors. No matter where you are in your cancer journey, I believe these six factors will give you hope as well. They are:

1. **A Positive Outlook**   4. **A Loving Family**
2. **Keeping Fit**   5. **Caring Friends**
3. **A Durable Faith**   6. **A Supportive Community**

Even if these six factors have not been a part of your life in the past, it's not too late to make constructive, healthy changes in your life. It's not too late to become the kind of person who not only survives but overcomes this disease. Cancer is a powerful adversary—but it's no match for those who have the optimism, character, faith, and courage to fight back.

So turn the page. Join me on my journey. Let's face cancer with optimism, hope, and courage. Let's stand together. Let's fight back.

Let's win.

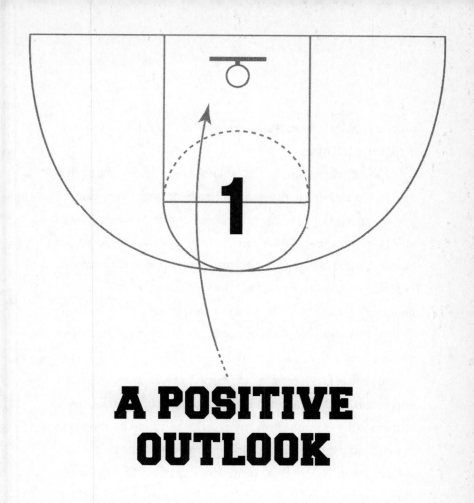

A POSITIVE OUTLOOK

The day Dr. Reynolds confirmed my cancer diagnosis, he told me that the first and most important factor in my favor was a positive, optimistic outlook. Even though Dr. Reynolds and I were just getting to know each other at that point, he knew my reputation well. He knew that I was a motivational writer and speaker, and that optimism is practically my trademark.

Up until the moment Dr. Reynolds confirmed that I did, in fact, have multiple myeloma, I had been able to operate on a kind of false optimism, otherwise known as denial. I was able to tell myself, *Cancer can't happen to me. Other people get cancer, but I've taken such good care of myself that it's unthinkable that I would ever get that disease. The blood work is wrong. Somebody made a mistake. This is nothing but a false alarm. It will be such a relief when Dr. Reynolds gives me the good news that I've got a clean bill of health after all.*

But once Dr. Reynolds explained my situation, directly and forthrightly, I no longer had the luxury of denial. I could still be optimistic, but now my optimism had to be rooted in reality and a clear-minded understanding of the facts.

The term "optimism" sometimes gets a bad rap in our culture today. Many people equate optimism with "wishing and hoping." Sometimes optimists are referred to as "Pollyannas," after the title character in a 1913 novel by Eleanor H. Porter and the 1960 Walt Disney movie by that name. If someone calls you a Pollyanna, it's probably not meant as a compliment. Cynical people use this term to portray optimists as foolishly cheerful, naive, and unable to accept reality.

But if you read Porter's novel *Pollyanna* or watch the Disney movie, you'll see that Pollyanna was not foolish or naive at all. She was an orphan who had experienced trials and losses, who constantly dealt with life's unfairness and with dour, nasty people, but she had learned to find hope and an optimal attitude in even the most hurtful situations.

> *"Cancer is a disease where the patient can contribute a great deal of help himself if he or she can retain their morale and their hopes."*
>
> —George Carman

If anyone wants to call me a Pollyanna, I will gladly accept the title. I believe it's a virtue and a strength to look for reasons to be glad and hopeful when you're going through trials and setbacks. There's no reason to believe that a pessimist or a cynic is any more realistic than a Pollyanna. In fact, I've always found that it is the Pollyannas, the optimists, who are the true realists, the achievers, the ones who get things done. We celebrate go-getting, positive-thinking optimists. After all, when was the last time you saw a statue honoring a pessimist?

In uncertain times, optimists always have the advantage. The optimist looks at his or her uncertain circumstances and says, "I don't really know how this is going to turn out, but I'm going to expect the best outcome and I'm going to work hard to make good things happen." By contrast, the pessimist looks at uncertain circumstances and says, "I'm always a victim of Murphy's Law—if something can go wrong, it will. I always have bad luck. Why even try? Might as well give up." Whether you are an optimist or a pessimist, your attitude frequently becomes a self-fulfilling prophecy.

Numerous scientific studies have shown a clear relationship between an optimistic mental attitude and the state of our physical and mental health. Optimists are statistically healthier people than pessimists with regard to such illnesses as clinical depression, heart disease, stroke, rheumatoid arthritis, fibromyalgia, and, yes, cancer. There are several obvious reasons for this, some having to do with the lifestyle of an optimist. Positive people tend to be more physically active, consume a more healthy diet, and do not feel the need to alter their moods with alcohol, drugs, and tobacco. Because optimists feel more confident and in control of their lives, they feel less stress in difficult situations—and emotional stress is known to play a role in depressing the immune system and other crucial systems in the body.

So when Dr. Reynolds told me that my optimism was going to help me in my battle with cancer, he was not just dispensing platitudes. He was giving me good medical advice. He was offering me a realistic assessment of some of the key factors in my medical prognosis. In my battle against cancer, he said, my positive mental attitude was one of my strongest allies. I latched on to this hope, and Dr. Reynolds's words have proven reliable again and again throughout my cancer journey.

That's why I want to pass this insight along to you: Make optimism your first ally. While there are no guarantees in any cancer battle, you have a realistic reason for optimism. Hold on to that hope. Maintain your optimism. Your positive attitude is going to get you through this.

> Hold on to that hope. Maintain your optimism. Your positive attitude is going to get you through this.

Aware of Our Influence

When Dr. Reynolds told me my optimism would aid me in my cancer battle, I couldn't comprehend what he meant. I was still in shock, and I couldn't fully grasp what he was telling me. It would take time for me to fully understand it. But just the fact that he was injecting hope at that time was a huge booster shot to my sagging morale.

During the shock of that moment, my head buzzed with questions: *Am I going to die from this disease? How long do I have to live? Am I going to feel horrible for the rest of my life? Am I even going to have a life, or am I going to become some sort of invalid?* I began to pour out these questions to Dr. Reynolds. I asked him what my life expectancy would be.

"Unless you go into remission," he said, "about two or three years. But if we can get you into remission, you can expect to live much longer. Some patients live for decades with myeloma. We're going to start a course of treatment that we believe has a very good chance of getting you into remission."

"What are my odds of remission?"

"With this course of treatment, I'd give you a seventy to seventy-five percent chance."

"Doctor, I like those odds."

And that became my initial basis for optimism. Yes, I was up against a tough opponent called *cancer*. But I had a realistic plan for attacking this opponent—and I had a realistic hope of remission.

Once I got past the initial shock and began entering the early stages of my treatment, I learned what the reality of this cancer battle was. I was introduced to all the different experiences a cancer patient goes through. Much of it was difficult. But a surprising number of experiences I had feared and avoided thinking about were not nearly as unpleasant as I had expected.

As I began to realize that I could handle everything that cancer was throwing at me, my optimism kicked into a higher gear. It's hard to maintain your optimism when you're facing many unknowns. But once the unknown becomes known, your optimism takes a giant leap skyward.

> *"The goal is to live a full, productive life even with all that ambiguity. No matter what happens, whether the cancer never flares up again or whether you die, the important thing is that the days that you have had you will have lived."*
>
> —Gilda Radner

I am a goal setter by nature. I set goals for each day, week, year, the next five years, and the next ten years. I want to achieve my life goals and accomplish my life's work. In order to do that, I need to stay strong and active, and to do that, I need to remain positive and upbeat. I have a natural advantage because optimism comes naturally to me—it's part of my character and personality.

But let's face it: cancer is a big-league opponent, a heavy hitter. In order to take on this challenge, I'm going to have to ramp up my optimism a lot. It's one thing to be an optimist when the sun is shining, the birds are singing, and everything is coming your way. It's quite another thing to be an optimist when the storm clouds close in around you and the wind is in your face.

I had written dozens of motivational books and given thousands of motivational speeches before I was diagnosed with cancer. But now we get to find out if all the things I've been writing about and speaking about for decades really apply in the toughest times of life.

Cancer is a major trial of adversity—one of the biggest. So, as we walk through this cancer journey, we have to ask ourselves, *Am I up to this challenge?* People are watching you and me. They want to see if we're going to stand firm in this crisis—or fall apart. The people around us will either be encouraged and inspired by the way we face our cancer battle—or they'll be disappointed and disillusioned.

I'm keenly aware that many of the people who have read my books or heard me speak are thinking, *Well, he had a positive message for going through good times, but it doesn't seem to hold water in tough times. I used to think Pat Williams had a lot to say, but when his values and principles were tested by adversity, he folded like a cheap suit.*

I am keenly aware of the influence I have. And I want you to be aware of the influence you have as well. We are all surrounded by people who closely watch the way we live our lives. They want to know if we walk the talk. Wherever I go, people are watching me—my children, my grand-children, the Orlando Magic family, and the people who hear me speak, read my books, or see me in the media. I don't want to let them down, so I'm fighting this battle and maintaining my optimism not just for myself but for them. And yes—for you.

You may have trouble believing what I'm about to say, but it's absolutely true: I don't really have any down moments. The worst moment of this whole cancer journey was when Dr. Reynolds confirmed the diagnosis. Since then, it has all been an upward climb, a journey of hope.

I attribute a lot of my optimism to the fact that I just don't have much time to sit and feel sorry for myself. I have an active travel and speaking schedule, I put in very full days at work, and when I get home from work, I know that I am about five hundred books behind in my reading. So I don't have time to sit and mope. I'm too busy living my life.

> I have an active travel and speaking schedule, I put in very full days at work, and when I get home from work, I know that I am about five hundred books behind in my reading. So I don't have time to sit and mope. I'm too busy living my life.

From the beginning of my cancer battle, Dr. Reynolds has advised me, "Pat, just live your life. We'll tuck the medical stuff around your life. We want you to live as much as possible the way you would live if you'd never had this diagnosis. When you're going about your job with the Magic, when you're speaking or writing, when you're with your children and grandchildren, do all the things you'd normally do. Don't cancel speaking engagements because you have a chemo session. We'll schedule the chemo around your speaking engagements."

And that is exactly what I've done.

Perpetual Optimism Is a Force Multiplier

At around the time that I was diagnosed, I was busy promoting my newly released book *Coach Wooden: The 7 Principles that Shaped His Life and Will Change Yours*—a book on the success secrets of the late, great Coach John Wooden. I sent copies of that book to a number of people, including legendary golfer Arnold Palmer.

Soon afterward, I received a wonderful letter from Arnold in which he referred to his own battle with prostate cancer. He wrote, "Pat, I understand you're going through a tough time right now. I wish you all the best with your treatment, and would only give you the same advice that people gave me when I was going through my ordeal: listen to what your doctors advise you and keep a positive attitude."

Every great victory in life begins with optimism and hope. In order to keep fighting against a determined enemy, we must believe that victory is possible, that our problems have a solution. This is especially true when the enemy we face is cancer.

During World War II, Winston Churchill rallied the people of Great Britain, summoning their courage and hard work through speeches that conveyed a tough-minded, realistic hope. Churchill didn't sugarcoat the sufferings that lay ahead of the British people. In his first speech as prime minister in 1940, he said, "I have nothing to offer but blood, toil, tears, and sweat. . . . What is our aim? . . . It is victory, victory at all costs, victory in spite of all terror, victory, however long and hard the road may be." The cancer battle is also a journey of blood, toil, tears, and sweat. The goal of that battle is victory at all costs—victory over cancer.

Dwight Eisenhower once said that having been through a number of military campaigns, he had often seen that in battle there comes a time when the enemy "looks fourteen feet tall and everyone takes alarm. But pessimism never won a battle." It's true. And this truth applies to cancer as well as to the battlefield. Sometimes this enemy seems bigger than we are—but pessimism never won a battle.

I don't want you to enter the battle of your life wearing rose-colored glasses. I want you to be *realistically* hopeful. I want you to face the challenges ahead armed with sound, reliable knowledge and a positive mental attitude. Whenever you face a major challenge in life, you must make a choice. You can choose to frame your problems as opportunities—or disasters.

Another military leader, General Colin Powell, once said, "Perpetual optimism is a force multiplier." This principle has been proven true countless times, both on the battlefield and in the battle against cancer. Optimism multiplies your strength and resources, increasing your advantage against your opponent. Optimism multiplies the effectiveness of your treatments and medications. Optimism magnifies the benefit you derive from exercise and a healthy diet.

If you choose to face cancer with a positive mental attitude, you will increase your odds of survival and victory over cancer. This doesn't mean that victory is guaranteed. Optimism is not magic, and a positive outlook is not a cure. But optimism attracts the forces in your life that help to make survival, life, hope, and victory much more likely.

"I took on cancer like I take on everything—like a mission and a job to accomplish."

—Sam Taylor-Wood

It's really only a matter of common sense. In every aspect of life, it is the optimists, not the pessimists, who are most likely to reach their goals. Optimists tend to be more proactive and decisive, because they expect their decisions to turn out right. Optimists tend to be more determined and persistent, because they believe their problems have solutions. Optimists don't waste time and energy on self-pity and resentment, because they believe that setbacks can be overcome. Optimists are more likely to cooperate with their treatment because they are confident they can bounce back from the adversity of cancer. And optimists tend to exhibit clearer thinking, a healthier immune system, and better digestive and heart health.

We all view life through the lens of our personality types, experiences, upbringing, joys, and disappointments. Some of us naturally find it easier to be optimistic than others. And let's face it: there are few experiences in life that can test your optimism more intensely than a battle with cancer. But the evidence is clear: an optimistic attitude can be as potent and healthful as good medicine.

In an online article for breast cancer patients, registered nurse Lucia Giuggio Carvalho and Dr. James A. Stewart discuss the emotional benefits of an optimistic mind-set:

> Having a positive attitude does not cure your breast cancer, but can make the journey more bearable. . . . Consider, for example, the pessimistic viewpoint—"Having breast cancer is overwhelming, I can't believe I have breast cancer"—versus an optimistic viewpoint—"I am living with breast cancer right now in my life and I am going to get through it." . . .
>
> To cultivate optimism and hope is to look at life differently. . . . Instead of your daily "things to do" list, keep a "gratitude" list. No matter what situation you find yourself in, there are people in your life, strengths and virtues you possess, for which you can exercise the spirit of gratitude.[3]

Double-blind clinical trials have shown that a positive attitude can actually enable cancer patients to experience a better prognosis and longer survival rates. One study, released in the March 2010 issue of the *Journal of Thoracic Oncology*, found that lung cancer patients who exhibited an optimistic outlook enjoyed a statistically significant survival advantage over their pessimistic counterparts. The patients in the study were scored according to the Optimism-Pessimism scale of the Minnesota Multiphasic Personality Inventory (MMPI). Patients of both sexes were classified as either optimistic or pessimistic personality types. The five-year survival rate for pessimists was 21.1 percent; the survival rate for optimists was 32.9 percent. This statistical relationship held true independent of such issues as cancer stage, medical treatment, smoking status, and so on. The single factor that seemed to have the greatest impact on survival was optimism.

One of the researchers who led the study, Paul Novotny, MS, of Mayo Clinic, said that this finding was so profound that it suggested that physicians should consider "cognitive therapy" (improving a patient's attitude and outlook) as a key aspect of patient care and treatment. While optimism is not a cure for cancer, a positive mental attitude clearly has medical and therapeutic benefits.[4]

A Realistic Optimist

I am realistic.
And I am optimistic.

I am realistic. And I am optimistic. The biggest challenge to my optimism is the fact that my form of cancer, multiple myeloma, is incurable. Most forms of cancer today are potentially curable, even when detected at an advanced stage. You will probably never hear a doctor pronounce a cancer patient "cured," even if the patient remains cancer-free for five years or more. In any individual case, there is always a chance of recurrence. Still, there are millions of people who have been treated for leukemia (cancer of the blood), or for cancer of the lungs, liver, or pancreas who have gone on to live cancer-free for decades. For now, however, multiple myeloma can't be cured. It must be constantly monitored, managed, and kept in remission through chemotherapy and other therapies.

Multiple myeloma is a cancer of the plasma cells (white blood cells) in the bone marrow. The blood is made of three kinds of cells: red cells that carry oxygen, platelets that cause blood to clot and stop bleeding, and plasma cells that produce antibodies to fight infection in the body. When those plasma cells begin to multiply too quickly and fail to shut off reproduction, they produce nonfunctioning antibodies called monoclonal proteins or paraproteins. These nonfunctioning antibodies are useless and do not fight infection. The first clue my doctors had that I had something wrong with my blood was when they found these useless antibodies (paraproteins) in my blood work.

These malfunctioning, rapidly multiplying plasma cells in the blood and marrow are myeloma cells. Doctors call a mass of myeloma cells a "solitary plasmacytoma." When multiple plasmacytomas are found, this is referred to as "multiple myeloma." Medical science still does not understand what causes plasma cells to become myeloma cells. All we know now is that once myeloma cells start reproducing out of control, they quickly crowd out other types of blood cells in the bone marrow.

Myeloma differs from most other cancers in that there is no cancer site in the body, no single tumor that can be removed. A surgeon may cut a tumor out of a patient's breast or colon, and if the cancer was confined to that site, there's a good chance that the cancer is now completely gone. But there's no myeloma tumor to remove. The myeloma is all throughout the bloodstream and bone marrow. As a nurse explained it to me, trying to take the cancer cells out of the blood and marrow would be like trying to take the sugar out of your coffee.

Though there's no cure, there's plenty of reason for optimism, because we are learning more and more about this disease all the time. Advances in treatment over the past few years have enabled many patients to live long, active, healthy lives.

"I keep dreaming of a future, a future
with a long and healthy life, not lived in
the shadow of cancer but in the light."

—Patrick Swayze

My friend Kathy Giusti, founder and CEO of the Multiple Myeloma Research Foundation (MMRF), was diagnosed with myeloma at age thirty-seven in the mid-1990s. At that time, the odds of surviving five years after the diagnosis were about 1 in 10. Worst of all, Kathy learned that there was virtually no research being conducted to develop new treatments for multiple myeloma. So, along with her twin sister, Karen, she founded the MMRF to raise funds for myeloma research and to develop new myeloma drugs. Today, the odds of surviving five years after a myeloma diagnosis have improved to about 4 in 10—and much of the credit for those improved odds goes to Kathy Giusti and the MMRF.

Kathy is an amazing myeloma success story herself, having lived with this disease for nearly two decades. In fact, the International Myeloma Foundation reports that approximately 100,000 Americans now live relatively normal lives in spite of a diagnosis of multiple myeloma. About 38 percent of patients with multiple myeloma live at least five years after the diagnosis, and 19 percent live at least ten years, and there are new therapies coming online all the time. Patients diagnosed today have good reason to hope that they may live even longer.

As medical science continues to develop a deeper understanding of all forms of cancer at the genetic and molecular level, the prospects for conquering cancer are rapidly increasing. Even patients with such pernicious cancers as lung cancer, pancreatic cancer, and brain cancer have reason to hope for a genuine cure within their lifetime.

The best hope for successful treatment of myeloma or any other cancer is early detection. In my own case, the myeloma was detected before many symptoms had presented themselves. The only symptom I was aware of prior to diagnosis was back pain. Bone pain is a common symptom of myeloma. But there are many other common problems that can cause back pain or bone pain, so when people go to the doctor complaining of these symptoms, the doctor often treats the symptoms a few times before performing a blood test and discovering the telltale signs of myeloma.

Myeloma weakens the bones, so bones tend to fracture more easily. Doctors sometimes suspect myeloma when a patient comes in with a fracture or other problem involving the bone.

People with myeloma often complain of a generalized feeling of exhaustion due to anemia. As the myeloma cells crowd out the red blood cells that carry oxygen throughout the body, the body no longer receives all the oxygen it needs. This causes the patient to feel anemic and tired.

Other symptoms can include mental confusion (caused by calcium in the blood due to myeloma breaking down calcium in the bones), loss of appetite, and nausea or vomiting. For some people, the first indication of myeloma is kidney failure, due to the inability of the kidneys to filter out high levels of paraproteins and calcium.

Any of these symptoms could occur in a person who does not have myeloma. So, if you experience any of these symptoms, don't assume you have myeloma. Instead, go to your doctor, explain your symptoms, and ask to be examined and tested.

If your doctor does all the tests and the results come back positive for myeloma, again, don't panic. Instead, realize that it's time for you to call upon your positive mental attitude. Listen carefully to your doctor. If at all possible, bring a friend, family member, or spouse. When your doctor is talking about your diagnosis, it's helpful to have someone with you who is a good listener, who asks good questions, and who takes good notes. I feel blessed that I had the foresight to bring Ruth to my appointment.

At this point, more than three years into my cancer battle, I feel optimistic about the future. Not wildly, irrationally optimistic. I know what I'm up against, and I am realistic about it. I'm in a battle for my life—but I have every reason to hope. Though I'm ready to die, I

> I feel optimistic about the future. Not wildly, irrationally optimistic. I know what I'm up against, and I am realistic about it. I'm in a battle for my life— but I have every reason to hope. Though I'm ready to die, I have every reason to go on with my life and to live it to the fullest.

have every reason to go on with my life and to live it to the fullest. Cancer is a factor in my life, but it doesn't own me.

That's what it means to be a realistic optimist.

An Optimist by Choice

Optimism is a choice—and it's a learnable skill. Even if you are not an upbeat and positive person by nature, it's not too late to change. You can retrain your mind to look at your life and your cancer in a new and optimistic way. When you do so, when you make a conscious choice to approach life with a positive mental attitude, you will increase your ability to fight this enemy—and you'll stack the odds of victory in your favor.

My friend and mentor Rich DeVos is co-owner of the Orlando Magic. Following his heart transplant in 1997, he wrote an encouraging book called *Hope from My Heart: 10 Lessons for Life*. He said this about an optimistic attitude:

If you expect something to turn out badly, it probably will. Pessimism is seldom disappointed. But the same principle also works in reverse. If you expect good things to happen, they usually do! There seems to be a natural cause-and-effect relationship between optimism and success. . . .

We can choose to laugh or cry, bless or curse. It's our decision: From which perspective do we want to view life? Will we look up in hope or down in despair?

> I believe in the upward look. . . . I am an optimist by choice as much as by nature.[5]

Rich DeVos is an optimist by choice, and so am I. You can be too. You can choose optimism, because optimism is an attitude choice. It's a habit of thinking. It's a learnable skill that we can build into our lives. Many people—and I number myself among them—have built a habit of optimism over a lifetime. In a world that seems to be divided between those who see the glass as half empty and those who see it as half full, I have always envisioned the glass as overflowing.

Some people, unfortunately, are not naturally optimistic. You may be a pessimist by nature and by force of habit. Perhaps you came from a family of pessimists, and you learned a can't-do attitude from your parents. Or perhaps life experiences have soured your outlook on life. For one reason or another, optimism just doesn't come naturally to you. If that's so, then it's time to change the way you think. Let me challenge you with a few ideas and suggestions for becoming a more optimistic person:

1. *Take time to focus intentionally on a positive attitude.* Take the next two months of your life and seriously devote yourself to becoming a person of optimism and having a positive outlook. Ask a few trusted friends to monitor your words and behavior, and

to point out to you the times when you sink into a pessimistic way of thinking. Become aware of the symptoms of a pessimistic mind-set. Pessimists tend to "horrible-ize" the events in their lives, turning every minor setback into a towering symbol of cosmic injustice: "Wouldn't you know it? The milk turned sour! My cornflakes are ruined! Why does everything happen to me?" Pessimists also tend to blame and berate themselves when things go wrong: "Why didn't I check the milk before I poured it on my cornflakes? How could I be so stupid?" Replace "horrible-izing" with optimizing. Learn to say, "Oh well, these things happen. I think I'll have some whole wheat toast and honey instead." Learn to isolate and minimize problems instead of blowing them up and making them bigger than life.

"Cancer can take away all of
my physical abilities. It cannot touch
my mind, it cannot touch my heart,
and it cannot touch my soul."

—Jim Valvano

---

2. *Read books of positive, motivational principles and quotations.* Feed your mind on optimistic thinking.

Read books (or listen to audiobooks) by positive thinkers like Norman Vincent Peale, Zig Zigler, John Maxwell, Brian Tracy, or, ahem, Pat Williams. Study the lives of people who overcame great obstacles and overwhelming odds to achieve great things (high-achieving people are invariably optimists). You will learn empowering, life-changing lessons by studying their lives.

3. *Surround yourself with optimistic sayings and positive music.* Write or print out motivational messages and post them where you will see them every day: your bathroom mirror, the dashboard of your car, the family message board, or the refrigerator door. Post encouraging Scripture verses. Carry optimistic quotations and Scripture passages in your wallet or put them on your computer, tablet, or smart phone. Load your iPod or other listening device with inspiring music, and listen to "positive, encouraging K-LOVE" on your FM radio (to find a K-LOVE station near you or to listen online, visit www.klove.com).

4. *Practice becoming a motivator and encourager to others.* It's impossible to be a pessimist while you are coaching others to be more positive. When you are with your spouse, kids, or fellow workers, practice lifting people up. Focus on helping other people to

feel positive, enthusiastic, and revved up. The best way I know to lift your own spirits is to become a cheerleader for others.

5. *Think rationally.* Sometimes people accuse optimists of being unrealistic, but I find that pessimists are generally far more unrealistic and irrational than optimists. People who sink into a pessimistic mood usually don't think clearly. If you feel pessimistic, you need to stop and think about *why* you feel that way. Your circumstances probably aren't any different now than they were yesterday when you felt optimistic. Upon reflection, you may realize that there's no rational basis for thinking negatively. Sure, you have cancer, but you are working with your doctors and it's under control. So make a decision that you're not going to let a momentary feeling of gloom darken your whole day. There's only one life per customer, so you'd better enjoy it while you have it. Why waste even a moment of your one and only irreplaceable life on irrational pessimism?

> There's only one life per customer, so you'd better enjoy it while you have it. Why waste even a moment of your one and only irreplaceable life on irrational pessimism?

6. *Meditate and pray.* We'll talk more about the spiritual response to cancer in Chapter 3. But for

now, let's acknowledge that meditation and prayer can play a huge role in shaping the way we think about our lives. If we are relaxed in mind and body, if we focus our thoughts outside ourselves and talk to God, and then listen to God speak to us within our innermost being, we can't help but develop a more positive, trusting, sacred awareness. As we invite the Spirit of God into our lives, our thoughts, and our emotions, we open ourselves to the most positive and life-affirming Force of all—the One who designed and created life.

7. *Maintain a journal.* Write down your thoughts, insights, and feelings of gratitude. It's okay to record those times when you're feeling sad or fearful—but remember to record your good experiences, joys, and accomplishments as well. Be sure to write down the reason why those good things happened. Later, you can read back over your journal—and you'll be amazed at how you have learned and grown through your cancer experience. On those occasions when you have an unhappy "valley" experience, be sure to write down the lessons you learn in the "valley." Those lessons will enable you to have more "mountaintop" experiences in the future.

If your spouse, loved one, or friend is going through a cancer battle, encourage him or her to adopt an optimistic mind-set. Don't expect that person to become an instant Pollyanna immediately after receiving a diagnosis. But gently, patiently encourage that person to choose optimism instead of bitterness, hope instead of resentment, and action instead of resignation. Wait for the right moment, when your loved one is in a receptive mood. Then offer a sensitive reminder that optimism is a health benefit that can give that person a much-needed edge in the cancer battle.

A Privilege, Not a Curse

When I started chemotherapy in February 2011, I would come into the chemo room at the Cancer Institute and I'd take my place in the chemo chair—a comfortable chair that looks a lot like a first-class airline seat. The doctors had installed a port in my upper chest so the chemo could be administered and blood could be taken directly from the port without sticking needles in my veins. I brought books and mail to read, and I used my cell phone to make calls. The chemo session would typically last three or four hours. After the first hour, I'd usually get sleepy. The next thing I knew, the nurse would be saying, "Mr. Williams, you've been napping for a few hours. You're all done." And I'd get out of the chair feeling refreshed.

At the beginning, my chemo sessions were rather impersonal. When I arrived for my first few sessions, I'd walk past the other chemo patients without saying anything, without an expression on my face, without really acknowledging my fellow cancer patients. The atmosphere in the room seemed gloomy and depressing.

One day, I arrived at the chemo room and a nurse took me aside. "Mr. Williams," she said, "the patients in the other chemo chairs know who you are and they know what you're going through. They're all going through a cancer battle, just as you are. There are a lot of sad people in that room. So from now on, when you come here, would you do these folks a favor? Would you greet them with a smile and give them a word of encouragement? If you'd do that before you start your chemo, I think it would give a big lift to the entire room—and it might even help people in their healing process."

I said, "I should have thought of that myself. Thanks for that suggestion."

From then on, whenever I went to the Cancer Institute for chemotherapy, I always entered the chemo room with a smile, some hugs, some high-fives, and a few words of optimism and hope. In the process of trying to spread some cheer, I've received a medicinal dose of happiness in return. I'm grateful to that nurse for reminding me that people are watching me at all times, and they want to know how I'm dealing with adversity. I have a responsibility to be a role model of optimism to everyone around me.

"When I found out I had cancer,
I just said one thing: 'I want to hold
on to life,' and that changed
everything for me."

—Scott Thompson

As you and I face our cancer battles, we need to continually think of others. We need to think of our influence and the legacy we're leaving to the people around us. Let's make an effort to always lift others up. We may not always feel like we're at our best. We may feel tired and anxious because of this battle we're fighting. We may just want to be left alone—but we shouldn't use our problems as an excuse to make others miserable. Let's keep encouraging others and living our lives as examples of the power of optimism.

When I was a catcher in the minor leagues, my manager in the Phillies farm system was former major league catcher Andy Seminick. He used to give us a pep talk when we were down a few runs and needed to fight back. I can still hear him say these words, followed by a splat of tobacco juice on the ground: "Grab yourself by the tail!"

Okay, I cleaned it up a bit. But he meant that when you're down, you need to pick yourself up. You need to get up off the ground, and even lift yourself by your own posterior if need be. Get back on your feet. Motivate yourself. Empower yourself. Talk yourself into a positive attitude. Convince yourself you can do it.

That's what I would say to anybody who is going through cancer and struggling to keep a positive attitude. Pick yourself up by the tail, get back on your feet, keep living your life, keep moving forward. You won't feel naturally optimistic every day. You won't feel like you used to before you had cancer. You won't feel 100 percent.

But let me tell you what I've found out: I am able to function pretty well at 80 percent. And sometimes I feel so encouraged that I'm able to notch it up to 90 percent. And that helps make up for those days when I feel like I'm at only 60 percent.

When I first heard that I had cancer, I went through a period of thinking, *Why me, Lord? What did I do to deserve this? What did I do to bring this on myself?* Well, that kind of thinking didn't last very long because it hit me that there are an awful lot of little kids in pediatric cancer wards. What did they do to deserve childhood leukemia or a childhood brain tumor? What did they do to bring this on themselves? Visit a pediatric cancer ward, and you'll see that those kids battle their cancers bravely and without complaint. Should we do any less?

There's a scourge that afflicts millions of people across our country and around the world. It's the scourge of cancer. There was a time when I didn't give much thought to cancer, but now I've been drafted into the anticancer army. I've been given an assignment. My mission is to make a difference in this battle against cancer.

I don't believe I've been cursed with cancer. I've been given a privilege. I would not have volunteered for this privilege, I assure you, but now that God has selected me for this honor, I am going to fight this battle against cancer with every weapon at my disposal.

> I don't believe I've been cursed with cancer.

And my first and most powerful weapon is an attitude of optimism.

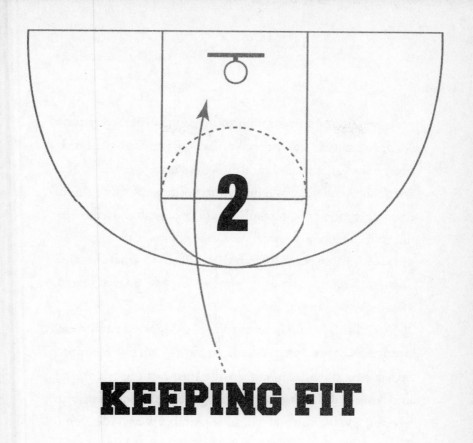

KEEPING FIT

I have nineteen children—four birth children, fourteen by international adoption, and one by remarriage. Audra Hollifield, the Orlando Magic's human resources director, has told me more than once that she's my twentieth kid. And I would be more than happy to adopt her and claim her as part of the Williams clan—especially since she quite probably saved my life.

It was Audra, after all, who arranged for all of the Orlando
Magic executives to undergo a daylong physical at Florida
Hospital's Celebration Health Assessment Center. In late
2010, she sent out a memo to the entire staff that said, in
essence, "Florida Hospital Celebration will call you to schedule your executive physical, and you will go." Of course, she
phrased it more politely than that, but that's what it boiled
down to. And to be honest with you, when I read that memo,
I was very unhappy.

Audra's office and mine are just a few doors down the hall
from each other, so as soon as I read the memo, I jumped
up, dashed down the hall, strode into her office without
knocking—and found her in the middle of a meeting with
her staff. With my usual tact and aplomb, I waved the memo
and said, "Aud, please tell me this is some kind of mistake!
I don't *really* have to take an entire day out of my schedule
just to get my blood siphoned and my temperature taken, do
I? I already went to my own doctor! I already had a physical!
I'm fine! I can skip this, can't I?"

Audra flashed me a serene smile worthy of the Buddha.
"Pat," she said, "they do an incredible job at Celebration.
They are very thorough. If you had to pay for this physical
out of your own pocket, it would probably cost you eight or
nine thousand dollars. But because it's part of our sponsor-
ship arrangement with Florida Hospital, you won't have to
pay anything out of pocket. It's practically a day at the spa.

Just go and enjoy yourself for the day. The people there are wonderful. You'll thank me for it."

I walked out of Audra's office huffing and puffing. I went back to my own office, gave the memo to my assistant, Andrew Herdliska, and had him make the appointment. I was sure of one thing—I was *not* going to thank Audra for making me waste a full day of my busy schedule getting probed and poked by people with needles, syringes, and rubber gloves.

As it turned out, of course, I could not have been more wrong. If Audra Hollifield had not sent me to the Celebration Health Assessment Center, I might not have been diagnosed until it was too late to save my life.

"People's view of cancer will change when they have their own relationship with cancer, which everyone will, at some point."

—Laura Linney

Audra recently reminded me of a conversation that she and I had had one day over lunch before my diagnosis. She remarked on the fact that I am an exercise fanatic, and that my home gym is better equipped than many professional gyms. She knew I had set goals for running in the Boston and New York City marathons on into my eighties, and that I was hoping to break the age records for those events. I worked out every day without fail. I'd lift weights, ride a stationary bike, and walk and run on the treadmill.

"Pat," she said, "it's unbelievable that with the schedule you have, you always manage to get in a full, daily workout. You never miss."

"Aud," I said, "do you know why I do that?"

"For your health?"

"For my old age," I said. "I'm preparing myself for when I'm old. If I don't prepare myself now, then when I'm seventy-five or eighty, it'll be too late. My body won't cooperate with me then. By exercising faithfully now, I make sure I don't suddenly discover it's too late to make up for lost time."

Audra and I had that conversation a year or two before I was diagnosed with cancer. After my diagnosis in January 2011, I realized I had been mistaken. My daily exercise regimen hadn't prepared me for old age. It had prepared me for my battle with cancer.

"Men, Don't Neglect Your Health"

The day Dr. Reynolds informed me of my diagnosis, he said, "The second factor in your favor is your good level of fitness. You exercise daily, you've kept trim and healthy, and you maintain a balanced diet. Your careful attention to staying fit and healthy is going to be a big advantage in your battle against cancer."

Dr. Reynolds okayed me to continue my normal travel, speaking, and writing schedule. Though the treatment regimen for multiple myeloma is not a walk in the park by any stretch of the imagination, it is easier to tolerate than many other cancer treatments. I took pills plus intravenous (IV) chemotherapy. One of the medications I received caused temporary hair loss, and all the medications left me feeling fatigued, but most did not cause nausea. So I was able to receive my treatments, then get right back to my regular schedule.

The doctor wanted me to continue exercising, but no more heavy workouts, no weight lifting, and no marathon training. I was glad I could continue working and exercising, because the physical and mental activity is therapeutic. If I had been forced to lie around in a hospital bed, I would have spent my days thinking about cancer and chemo—and that's no way to live. My commitment to keeping physically fit was a key factor in my treatment and recovery.

If I had been forced to lie around in a hospital bed, I would have spent my days thinking about cancer and chemo—and that's no way to live. My commitment to keeping physically fit was a key factor in my treatment and recovery.

I had known that two of my baseball heroes, longtime Yankees pitcher Mel Stottlemyre and former American League power hitter Don Baylor, had been diagnosed years earlier with some sort of cancer. But only when I was diagnosed with multiple myeloma did I realize that they had received the same diagnosis I had. Stottlemyre was a pitching coach with the Yankees when he was diagnosed with myeloma in 1999, and his doctors told him he had about three years to live. Almost fifteen years later, Stottlemyre is still in remission. And Don Baylor, who was the Mets' bench coach when he was diagnosed in 2003, also remains in remission.

These two athletes were both in good physical condition when they were diagnosed. Perhaps their own focus on fitness had a significant impact on their ability to live with myeloma many years beyond what their doctors predicted. Mel Stottlemyre and Don Baylor gave me hope that I, too, could beat the odds and beat this cancer. I might even be able to remain in remission until medical science finds a lasting cure.

After I was diagnosed, I wondered how I would break this news to my nineteen children, my friends and colleagues in the Magic organization, and the Orlando community. I was inclined to keep the news within the family for a while, but Dr. Reynolds recommended that I get the news out sooner rather than later. He pointed out how hard it would be to keep this matter a secret, especially with nineteen children in the family, most of whom are active on Facebook and other social media.

"My suggestion," Dr. Reynolds said, "is that you gather the media and make a public announcement. That way, you can make sure the information is reported accurately instead of being distorted by rumors."

That made sense to me, so I contacted Joel Glass, the Orlando Magic's media director, and he made the arrangements. We held the press conference in mid-February, and Dr. Reynolds was at my side. I had just started twice-weekly chemotherapy sessions, so I was feeling physically tired going into that event. I asked God for the strength to deliver an important message to the Orlando community and the national sports community—a message of hope and faith. As the lights came on and I was introduced, I felt God's strength flowing into me.

I began with the announcement that I had been diagnosed with multiple myeloma, then I turned it over to Dr. Reynolds. He took the roomful of reporters to med school, telling them exactly what multiple myeloma is and how he and his medical team planned to treat it. "Myeloma is not a curable disease," he explained, "but it is treatable. Our goal is to keep Pat in remission. I expect him to be able to live with this for many years. Twenty years ago, people diagnosed with myeloma faced a death sentence. But with treatments available today, patients commonly live for many years—and those treatments are improving all the time." He added that myeloma research, like research into most cancers, is tragically underfunded and needs more support.

After Dr. Reynolds had finished his explanation, I talked about my plans for the future. "I'm going to beat this," I said. "I'm fully engaged with the activities that bring me joy and fulfillment. I'm going to continue to play an active role in the Orlando Magic organization and in the Orlando community. I don't think you want me to sit around sucking my thumb and bemoaning my problems. So I intend to go on with my life as normally as I'm able. The chemotherapy does make me tired, so I'm sleeping a little more than I used to. But I'm not having any serious reactions to the chemo."

> *"Men [need to] be more aware*
> *about prostate cancer and*
> *their health in general."*
>
> —Herbie Mann

I had a special message for men. "We men tend to be driven and always on the go," I said, "and that means we often put our own health last. When I was told I needed to go in for a checkup, I didn't want to take the time away from my busy schedule. I was sure I was in fine shape and didn't need to waste my time in the doctor's office. But the doctors found a problem in my blood work—and that's how the myeloma was discovered. If I hadn't gone in for that checkup, who knows when I would have been diagnosed. By then, it might have been too late. So men, don't neglect your health. Take care of yourself. Get regular checkups."

I also talked about how my faith was carrying me through this crisis. "When I was diagnosed," I said, "I had a decision to make. I could turn my back on God and write him off—or I could climb up into his lap, reach up and hug him by the neck as hard as I could, and not let go. I have elected to do the latter. I've always felt there was one more chapter left in my life, a grand finale. Perhaps that is what we're seeing now. I'm being called to a new ministry of hope and help to others."

Ruth and about half of our brood of adult children were also with me at the press conference. As we were about to conclude, I removed my blazer to reveal the Magic blue T-shirt underneath. Lettered across the front of the shirt was my new slogan, THE MISSION IS REMISSION. Ruth and the kids also wore matching T-shirts—and the slogan was greeted with cheers and applause.

Breaking the Rules

Is it possible to take a mania for fitness to an unhealthy extreme? Well, if anyone could do it, I could. And I did.

Dr. Reynolds warned me that having been diagnosed with multiple myeloma, I needed to be very careful with my bones. He told me, "The *sine qua non* of myeloma is that it weakens the bones and can actually cause bones to break." While I was pondering the meaning of *"sine qua non,"* he added, "When I was in training, a young serviceman, a paratrooper, came in with injuries from making his first parachute jump. It should have been a routine jump, but when he landed, he broke multiple bones in his legs. That was how he found out he had multiple myeloma—his bones were weakened by the disease, and they snapped like kindling when he hit the ground."

The doctor told me that story for a reason. He was giving me my marching orders and trying to impress upon me the importance of not putting any extra stress on my bones, especially my back. In retrospect, I realize he was trying very hard to get my attention, because he tried to say it several different ways. But I have to admit that while Dr. Reynolds was telling me I needed to be extra careful, I was mentally thinking of exceptions, work-arounds, and rationales that would enable me to continue exercising the way I wanted to.

I was resigned to the fact that I wouldn't be running marathons—at least, not for a while. I agreed to scale back my weight lifting—a bit. As for his paratrooper story—well, I had no immediate plans to be jumping out of airplanes, so

I sort of blew it off. I nodded and said, "Sure, Doc, sure—I'll be careful."

So I got back into my daily schedule of traveling and speaking, my duties at the office, and my exercise routine. At first, I treated my back rather gingerly because I still had back pain as a reminder of the disease in my bone marrow. But as the chemotherapy and oral medications took effect, my back pain subsided. Dr. Reynolds warned me that even if I was feeling better, I should not forget to follow doctor's orders. He told me the stationary bike was a no-no, because it would put too much strain on my backbone.

But as I began feeling better, I gained confidence that I could put more stress on my back. I reasoned that if my back felt better, then it must be getting stronger. About two or three weeks after the press conference, I was on my exercise bike, pedaling like I had before the diagnosis. I felt good, I felt strong, I felt like my old self again—until suddenly, I felt the most incredible pain imaginable.

> I felt good, I felt strong, I felt like my old self again—until suddenly, I felt the most incredible pain imaginable.

I rolled off the bike, slumped to the floor, and lay there writhing and groaning. Ruth found me and immediately called Dr. Reynolds. The doctor told her to call for an ambulance. He was putting me in the hospital.

At the hospital, they x-rayed my back. The pictures showed that I had fractured one of the vertebrae in my back. It was a compression fracture, the result of putting too much strain on my backbone while exercising—exactly what Dr. Reynolds had warned against. There was a great deal of swelling around the fracture, plus a few other complications.

A neuroradiologist at the hospital performed a procedure called a vertebroplasty, which entailed injecting a substance into the compressed bone, causing it to re-expand and remove the pressure from my nerves. The result was amazing. The procedure immediately alleviated my back pain and helped to restore the integrity of my spine.

After the procedure, they put me in a hospital bed—the first time in my life I had ever been hospitalized. I had a fever and I was having a little trouble breathing. But I had a bigger problem, and when Dr. Reynolds came in to see me, I told him about it.

"Doc," I said, "I have to be out of here by morning."

He chuckled. He thought I was kidding.

"I'm serious," I said. "I'm scheduled to give a talk tomorrow morning at the Convention Center. Two thousand people are going to be sitting in their seats, waiting for me to come out and give a speech. It's too late for me to cancel. I have to be there."

"Pat," he said, "you've just had back surgery. You're in no condition to give a speech. You're in no condition to get out of that bed."

I've been a salesman all my life. I honestly believe I could sell Kryptonite to Superman. But selling Dr. Reynolds on the idea of letting me out of that hospital to give a speech took all the persuasion and salesmanship I could muster. To this day, I'll bet Dr. Reynolds wonders how I talked him into that—but he reluctantly agreed.

I had undergone back surgery at 6:00 PM, was transferred to a hospital room at 8:00 PM, and had an oxygen mask over my face and beeping monitors strapped to my body. Because of the swelling in my back, Dr. Reynolds gave me a powerful diuretic—and that daggone little pill had me dashing to the bathroom all night. By morning, I had lost several pounds of water weight.

It was a rough night and I got very little sleep—but by 5:30 AM, when the nurse came in to check on me, I was shaved, dressed, and ready for showtime. I had made transportation arrangements with Ruth and Andrew, and I was good to go.

Dr. Reynolds came by before I left, and I could see the surprise on his face. I'm sure I looked like a completely different person from the pain-racked invalid who had needed emergency back surgery the previous day. I felt physically weak from the ordeal and from lack of sleep, and I knew I wouldn't be able to deliver that speech standing up. But I was emotionally energized, and I knew I'd do fine if I could deliver it sitting down, much as Coach John Wooden delivered his speeches in his later years.

I didn't need the oxygen mask anymore—I was breathing just fine. But I could see the anxious expression on Dr. Reynolds's face. He undoubtedly expected to get a call in a couple of hours, informing him that his patient had collapsed onstage. But the worry in Dr. Reynolds's eyes was more than offset by the determination in my eyes. I thanked him for his support and for all he had done to nurse me back to some semblance of health.

"Every day I challenge this cancer and survive is a victory for me."

—Ingrid Bergman

Ruth picked me up in the car and drove me to the Convention Center. Andrew was in the parking lot with a golf cart, ready to take me to the speaking engagement. When it was time for my speech, they brought me onstage in a wheelchair—the first time in my life I had ever sat in a wheelchair, much less delivered a speech from one.

The audience and I had a great time together. It went very well. They were appreciative, and I came away feeling energized.

That experience was a lesson for me. I found out that I needed to take doctors' orders a little more seriously. I'm not saying I became a model patient and that I always did what my doctor told me—who are we trying to kid? But it really hit home to me that I had almost missed a speaking engagement because I had failed to obey Dr. Reynolds's orders about exercise bikes.

From then on, whenever Dr. Reynolds would lay down the rules he wanted me to follow, I was careful not to break them—I'd bend them only a little.

"Mission Accomplished!"

One benefit of running marathons is that they teach powerful, unforgettable lessons in perseverance and endurance. In every one of the fifty-eight marathons I've run, without exception, I've reached a point where my body and soul screamed, "Quit!"—yet something within my spirit said, "Keep going!" Each time my persevering spirit drove me on to the finish line, I learned a little more about what it means to fight on against adversity, pain, and exhaustion.

Throughout my marathon career, the words of the apostle Paul have spoken to me, motivated me, and kept me in the running: "Do you not know that in a race all the runners run, but only one gets the prize? Run in such a way as to get the prize. Everyone who competes in the games goes into strict training. They do it to get a crown that will not last, but we do it to get a crown that will last forever. Therefore

I do not run like someone running aimlessly; I do not fight like a boxer beating the air. No, I strike a blow to my body and make it my slave so that after I have preached to others, I myself will not be disqualified for the prize" (1 Corinthians 9:24–27).

> I don't run marathons anymore—doctor's orders. So I've made this cancer battle my new marathon, my long-distance race against cancer.

I don't run marathons anymore—doctor's orders. So I've made this cancer battle my new marathon, my long-distance race against cancer. And I'm finding that those fifty-eight marathons I ran over the past fifteen years have turned out to be the best preparation anyone could undergo for a cancer battle. In fact, marathon running prepared me in ways I never foresaw or imagined.

When Dr. Reynolds told me I had myeloma, he also told me I had a 70–75 percent chance of remission with the help of chemotherapy. Those sounded like good odds and I was encouraged. Immediately I came up with the slogan we announced at the press conference: THE MISSION IS REMISSION.

Soon after the press conference, I was asked to speak to a group of executives for a national restaurant chain. When I arrived for the event, they unveiled a huge banner that read THE MISSION IS REMISSION. All of the participants at the event signed the banner, and they gave it to me to take home.

Arriving home, I showed it to Ruth, and she put it up in the living room. As soon as you walked in the front door, you would see that huge banner, a powerful reminder of my goal.

After I began chemotherapy, it soon became clear that the treatments weren't working as well as Dr. Reynolds had hoped. He explained to me that when you give the same treatment to several patients, some patients respond well, others not so well. In my case, the myeloma was responding partially to the chemotherapy, but not dramatically enough.

My friend Kathy Giusti of the MMRF explained one possible reason why people respond differently to the same treatments. "Myeloma, like most cancers," she said, "is very heterogeneous. There is not one type of myeloma. There are more like ten types. Pat, your myeloma is completely different from my myeloma, which is completely different from Mel Stottlemyre's myeloma. We all have different types of the disease."

As a result, a cancer drug that works wonders for Kathy may have almost no effect on my myeloma. That's why the MMRF is actively engaged in finding new ways to analyze and understand cancer cells at the genomic level, so that we can better develop and target drugs to work against each specific form of myeloma.

When I was being treated in 2011, my doctors didn't have this kind of information to work with in targeting my cancer. The medical team pumped several different drugs into me, trying to bring my numbers down for the better part of a year, but the cancer proved to be a stubborn opponent. My doctors couldn't get me into remission. I was up against the Babe Ruth of cancers—so I told them (in baseball terms) that I wanted them to give me their "out" pitch, the pitch they could always count on to get the batter out. I told the doctors to empty the medicine cabinet and throw it all at me.

So Dr. Reynolds referred me to Dr. Yasser Khaled, a multiple myeloma and stem cell transplant specialist at Florida Hospital. It was Dr. Khaled who ultimately harvested about 4.9 million healthy stem cells from my bloodstream.

"In terms of fitness and battling through cancer, exercise helps you stay strong physically and mentally."

—Grete Waitz

The stem cell harvesting procedure wasn't particularly painful, but it was tedious and uncomfortable. The doctors gave me shots to stimulate the stem cells and get them moving through my bloodstream, so that they could be caught and filtered. They inserted three tubes into my chest—an arrangement called a Hickman TriFusion catheter. My entire blood system passed through those tubes and into the machine, which filtered out my stem cells. Then the blood was recycled back into my body. I could see the stem cell material as it accumulated in a plastic bag.

The harvested stem cells were placed in frozen storage. Once the stem cells were harvested, Dr. Khaled's team gave me a massive blast of chemo to kill the remaining cancer cells in my bone marrow. And I do mean it was a *massive* chemo blast. The chemo was administered in two sessions in late 2011, and each session lasted ninety-six hours.

My doctors tried to explain to me in medical terms what they were doing to me, but it was my nurse, Nancy, who broke it down into terms I could understand. "It's like a farmer with his field," she said. "He plows the soil and prepares it to be a rich treasure of good soil. He's trying to get the soil just right so that it will be good for the seeds, so the crop can grow strong and healthy. The soil is your bone marrow, the seeds are your stem cells, and the crop will be healthy new bone marrow without cancer. Good seed going back into good soil will make you strong and healthy."

Finally, they thawed out the healthy stem cells and infused them back into my body. There, the cells multiplied and produced healthy new blood cells. The process of transplanting the stem cells required eleven large syringes attached to outlets on the TriFusion tubing. It was an all-day process, but painless. I slept through most of it.

The healthy stem cells grafted and multiplied. Within days of the transplant procedure, the doctors informed me that I was finally in remission. Soon after getting that good news, I came home and was surprised to discover that Ruth had taken down the huge THE MISSION IS REMISSION banner. In its place was a new banner that read MISSION ACCOMPLISHED! I had a lot to be thankful for, and a lot to celebrate. I had just made it through the toughest year of my life. God, working in concert with my doctors and the prayers of so many family members and friends, had produced a miracle in my life.

I now have three birthdays to celebrate every year: my physical birthday on May 3, 1940; my spiritual birthday (the day I committed my life to God) on February 22, 1968; and my remission birthday of February 10, 2012. I plan to celebrate each of my three birthdays with a big party, surrounded by my family and friends.

Please understand—being in remission does not mean I'm cured. I still have multiple myeloma. As Dr. Reynolds told me, "Our goal is to keep you healthy and in remission for as long as we can. There are new technologies coming along all the time. Almost every day, I hear about some brand-new approach to treating cancer—and some of them are just a few years from being approved for use. The longer you keep going, Pat, the greater the odds you will benefit from one of these exciting new discoveries."

Competing Against Cancer

It's a miracle that you are reading these words right now, because it's a miracle I am here to write them. I had missed the cutoff age for the stem cell transplant procedure that saved my life. My doctors simply will not consider performing a stem cell transplant on someone who is older than sixty-five. I was seventy-one. Why did the doctors waive the age limitation in my case?

> It's a miracle that you are reading these words right now, because it's a miracle I am here to write them.

There is only one reason: I had kept myself in excellent physical condition. I had always worked out daily, run marathons, paid careful attention to my fitness and nutrition, and had avoided alcohol and tobacco. I had taken care of my health because I wanted to be in good physical condition throughout my life and on into old age. But, as it turned out, that intense, daily focus on physical fitness also paid off by earning me an exemption from the age sixty-five cutoff policy for stem cell transplants.

That policy is not arbitrary, cruel, or designed to favor the young over the old. In fact, even a person who is young will probably be rejected as a candidate for stem cell transplant if he or she has poor overall health and fitness. It's simply a matter of the most realistic allocation of medical resources. The stem cell transplant procedure takes a serious toll on the cardiovascular system. If you know that the procedure is likely to kill your patient through a heart attack or stroke, it makes no sense to do the procedure.

So there I was, turning seventy-one, having passed the cutoff age six years earlier, yet the chemotherapy just wasn't working. Without a stem cell transplant, I faced a death sentence. But even with the transplant procedure, there were no guarantees that it would put me in remission, or even that I would survive the stress of the procedure. I wondered if the stem cell transplant was just a last-ditch effort with little hope of success.

So I asked Dr. Khaled, "How many stem cell transplants have you done?"

"Three hundred."

"How many have been successful?"

"Three hundred."

"Wait a minute—are you telling me your success rate is one hundred percent?"

"That's exactly what I'm telling you."

"How in the world do you have a perfect record?"

"I choose my patients very carefully."

And remember, Dr. Khaled is not just thinking of maintaining a perfect record. He is thinking of his patients first. He will choose a course of treatment that is most likely to extend the life span and the quality of life of his patient. If he doesn't consider you a candidate for stem cell transplant, it's not because he's concerned about his box score. It's because he's concerned about his patients. He doesn't want to perform a procedure that is likely to end a patient's life.

You and I bear the responsibility for our own lives and our own health. The doctor is there to diagnose our ills, bind our wounds, prescribe medications for our diseases, and so forth—but the doctor can't make our daily exercise decisions and nutritional choices. If you are overweight and out of shape, if you abuse your body with drugs and alcohol and too many doughnuts and ice cream sundaes, you can't blame your doctor for withholding a medical procedure that would be as likely to kill you as save you, given the general state of your health. If you are running on fumes, if you've spent a lifetime as an overeating couch potato, it's not the doctor's fault that you are not a good candidate for a stem cell transplant.

*"Nothing I did contributed to
me having cancer, so I can't sit back
and say, 'Oh why me.' Why not me?
Why does tragedy always have
to hit someone else?"*

—Eric Davis

My advice to you, whether you are currently a cancer patient or you want to prepare for a possible cancer battle in the future, is that you start right now becoming as healthy as you can possibly be. You can't immediately reverse decades of neglecting your health, but don't let that stop you from doing what you can. You can begin eating a heart-healthy diet that is high in protein and fiber and low in saturated fats and carbohydrates. I'm not saying you should "go on a diet." I'm saying you should make *permanent* lifestyle changes that will enable you to become fit and healthy for the rest of your life. Join a gym or just get out and walk.

If you are not a cancer patient yet, remember: 1 out of 2 men and 1 out of 3 women will face cancer in their lifetime. Don't wait. Tennessee Titans wide receiver Nate Washington has a great slogan—"Stay ready so you don't have to get ready"—and I think his words apply to health and cancer preparedness as well as to football. Start preparing *now*, get healthy *now*, and stay ready so you won't have to get ready for a cancer battle in the future.

And if you are already a cancer patient, eating a heart-healthy diet is going to weigh heavily in your favor. It's not too late to start eating a healthy diet and treating your body to the exercise it needs. Wherever you are, whatever your age, whatever the status of your health right now, start getting yourself in shape for the battles ahead.

When I was exercising and watching my nutrition during my youth and middle-aged years, I thought I was getting in shape so I could keep up with my children and grandchildren. And that's reason enough to stay in shape. But now I have to add that I've been getting in shape for my cancer battle. Cancer is the ultimate opponent, and a cancer battle is the ultimate marathon. Though I didn't always realize it, I've been in this race all my life, and I am still in it to win. I've always hated to lose, so I'm competing hard against cancer.

Before I began the stem cell transplant, I asked Dr. Reynolds, "What's the shortest hospital stay anyone has had after a stem cell transplant?"

"Twelve days," he said.

"Doc, I'm going to break that record. I have to get out to speak at a Boy Scout event."

"We're not concerned with breaking records, Pat. Dr. Khaled and I have just one concern, and that's to get you healthy and functioning again so you can go on about your life and your speaking schedule."

I listened to what Dr. Reynolds told me, and I fully understood that they weren't interested in breaking records.

> I'm a competitor, and I always enjoy a competitive challenge. I knew that the best way for me to recover from the stem cell transplant was to look upon it as an athletic challenge—and to view myself as an athlete seeking to break the record.

But I'm a competitor, and I always enjoy a competitive challenge. I knew that the best way for me to recover from the
stem cell transplant was to look upon it as an athletic challenge—and to view myself as an athlete seeking to break
the record.

Not long before the transplant procedure, Kathy Giusti of
MMRF called me and told me that her organization wanted
to honor me at an annual sports-related event the foundation held in Chicago every year. Well, I was touched—and
with my ties to the Windy City (I was general manager of
the Chicago Bulls from 1969 to 1973), I eagerly accepted.

But Kathy did have a concern about the timing of the
event. She said, "Pat, I think you should think it over before
saying yes. The event takes place just a couple of weeks after
your stem cell transplant. I've had a stem cell transplant
myself, so I know how much they take out of you. We'd like
to have you at this event, but I want you to know that it's okay
if you can't do it because it's too soon after your procedure."

I had to laugh because she sounded so worried about me.
I said, "Kathy, are you kidding? I've got a whole book tour
scheduled before that!"

"A book tour!"

"Yes, Dr. Reynolds promised that he could time the transplant to coincide with my speaking and travel schedule. It
looks like the transplant is going to dovetail nicely with
everything I have on the docket."

"Pat, a stem cell transplant is a really hard procedure. I'm afraid you're moving too fast, trying to do too much."

I said, "Kath, it's gonna be fine. It's gonna be just fine."

And it was fine. I had the stem cell transplant, followed by a time of recuperation in the hospital. And just as I had planned, I beat the record. The old record was twelve days; I was out in ten. Dr. Reynolds just shook his head.

I held a press conference the day I came out of the hospital, because I wanted the community to see that I was competing hard against this cancer. I wanted to give people hope, and I wanted to spread the word that cancer can be beaten. It takes optimism, toughness, and a competitive spirit, but we can beat this thing. I also wanted people to know that we need more research, and that means we need people who are willing to step up and donate to the cause of finding a cure.

My book tour went well, and I went to Chicago and we had a great evening. I spoke at the event, Kathy and the MMRF recognized me for the work I was doing to raise awareness of myeloma research, and my daughter Karyn, who is a Nashville recording artist, got up on the stage with me, sang to me, and made me proud. It was unforgettable.

How about you? Are you a competitor? Do you have what it takes to take on this opponent called cancer and fight back? Don't give in. Don't surrender. People are watching you, counting on you, and they want to know how much fight there is in you. Don't let them down. Don't let yourself down.

Fight hard.

Fight Cancer with Knowledge

On Thanksgiving Day 2011, I was in the hospital undergoing a round of intensive chemo in preparation for my stem cell transplant. Audra Hollifield came to the hospital to visit me. Ruth was there, too. The three of us chatted together for a bit, then I said, "Hey, Aud, let me show you around the place." It was a special unit for chemo patients and it was furnished with all the latest high-tech medical equipment. In fact, the place looked like a set from *Star Trek*.

Audra said, "Okay, Pat, give me the tour."

So I grabbed my IV stand—I had a tube attached to me—and I pulled the stand along with me. Ruth, Audra, and I went up and down the hallway, pausing to look in some of the rooms. We stopped at the nurses' station, and I introduced Audra to my caregivers. Then I showed Audra the exercise room. I pulled my IV stand up next to the treadmill, climbed up, turned it on, and started walking at a brisk pace.

I noticed Ruth and Audra talking to each other while I exercised. It wasn't until weeks later that I discovered what they were talking about: me. For some reason, they thought it was odd that I would be exercising in a hospital. Apparently, when you're in a hospital, you're expected to lie down and rest.

Well, I always thought a hospital was a place to get healthy! How are you supposed to get well by lying on your back all day? If you want to get healthy, you've got to get up and *move*! You've got to get your blood circulating, your heart pumping, your lungs expanding, and your muscles in motion. A hospital stay is no excuse for dogging it.

"I don't eat fast food any more,
not since I got cancer."

—Paul Henderson

Okay, if your doctor tells you to stay in bed, then follow doctor's orders. But if your doctor clears you to move around, then get active! Even if you have cancer, get as fit as you can. Whether you are at home or in the hospital, take time to exercise. Discipline your body and your soul, so that you will be in top condition for fighting this cancer battle.

When Dr. Reynolds told me I had cancer, he also told me, "I don't want you to go home and sit around the house and mope. I don't want you to spend the rest of your life focused on cancer. I want you to be fully engaged in your normal life. Obviously, there are a few things you have to give up, like running marathons and catching at an old-timers' baseball game. But your work, your speaking, your writing, your travel, all of that can continue pretty much as it did before you had cancer. You can even exercise, as long as you don't put too much stress on your bones, especially your spine."

Dr. Reynolds even cleared me to get back on the exercise bike, which has been a lifesaver for me. Because of the large amounts of chemotherapy I've undergone, my feet are plagued with neuropathy—damage to the peripheral nerves. The neuropathy makes it impossible for me to run or jog right now, but I can handle a workout on the stationary bike, no problem. I have light weights that I work out with, and I've been able to stay reasonably fit in spite of the steroids I take, which tend to produce weight gain.

Whether you're a cancer patient, the loved one of a cancer patient, or you simply want to prepare yourself for a possible cancer battle in the future, I want to challenge you. I want to encourage you to take a few simple steps to improve your health and your fitness level so you will be better equipped to fight this opponent called cancer.

Step 1: Maintain a Focus on Healthy Diet and Exercise

Some people, after receiving a cancer diagnosis, give up on their health. They say to themselves, *Oh, what's the use? Why bother to stay fit? Why waste time and energy exercising?*

I have cancer, so I guess my exercising days are over. Nonsense! Now is when you need a fit and healthy body more than ever.

Poor diet, obesity, and lack of physical activity are factors in the development of many types of cancer and in many cancer deaths. Physical inactivity not only leads to increased body weight but also harmful effects on the endocrine system (the system of glands that produce vital hormones) and the immune system (which protects the body from disease).

In most cases (unless your doctor tells you otherwise), you don't need a radically restricted diet. A cancer-fighting diet is generally a basic heart-healthy diet—a diet high in vegetables, fruits, whole grains, and low-fat protein sources (such as white meat chicken or turkey), and low in salt, sugar, saturated fat, processed meats, and red meats. Following a heart-healthy diet on a continual, lifestyle basis is one of the best things you can do to prevent cancer—or to fight cancer if you've been diagnosed.

> Following a heart-healthy diet on a continual, lifestyle basis is one of the best things you can do to prevent cancer—or to fight cancer if you've been diagnosed.

Step 2: Build Relationships with Your Healthcare Team

When I was undergoing chemotherapy, being treated for my compression fracture, or receiving my stem cell transplant, I made it a point to get to know my caregivers on a first-name basis. I enjoyed making conversation with the nurses, finding out about their families, and discovering who they were as people. I have always been fascinated with people and their stories. But when those people are taking care of me, and helping to improve my health and quality of life, I feel a special connection to them.

It's not that I want to receive any special treatment from them. I just happen to think that when my health and my life are on the line, I would much rather be cared for by friends than by strangers. And I like to think that they feel they are not just monitoring vital signs and injecting foods into tubes, but they are taking care of a good friend, someone they know personally, someone who knows them.

Throughout this cancer battle, I have felt personally bonded with a number of special people. One of those special relationships was with Dr. Robert Reynolds himself. Even before I came to him for treatment, he was an Orlando Magic season ticket holder. Long before he was my doctor, he was one of the many valued Magic fans who fill our arena. Now when I go to a Magic game, I can look up into the stands and spot Dr. Reynolds in an instant. He's the friendly face I've gotten to know so well, and he and his wife are always seated in the same spot, wearing their Magic blue T-shirts with the white lettering that reads THE MISSION IS REMISSION. He's one of my biggest fans and supporters—and the feeling is fondly mutual.

And there's Dr. Khaled. Unfortunately, Dr. Khaled, my stem cell transplant specialist, is not a Magic fan. Oh, he loves NBA basketball, but for reasons that are completely beyond my comprehension, he's a fan of (it pains me to say it!) the New York Knicks! I rarely visit him without giving him a jab about it—and he jabs me right back! But I love this man, and he knows it. I might not be here today if not for his compassion and his healing skills.

Step 3: Maintain as Normal a Life as Possible

One of the best things I had going for me once I got out of the hospital was that my assistant, Andrew, helped me maintain my normal schedule and routines. For years, he has been setting up my speaking schedule, arranging my travel, and making sure I knew where I had to go and when I had to be there. After my cancer diagnosis, he didn't baby me or coddle me. He kept me focused and on-task. I needed that. If he had treated me like a semi-invalid, I might have lapsed into that role. Instead, Andrew always treated me the same as he always had. He helped keep my life structured and moving forward.

---

*"Life is a terminal condition.
We're all going to die. Cancer patients
just have more information."*

—Kris Carr

Andrew once explained how he felt at the time. "I felt terrible," he said. "My boss had cancer, and you never know about cancer. It's a serious curveball, and I didn't want to pile the stress of his daily workload on top of the stress of the cancer. But at the same time, Pat doesn't want to be treated like a cancer patient. He needed positive energy around him. He needed to feel normal. He needed to live productively, in spite of the chemo and stem cell transplants and everything else that was going on medically. So my job was to keep things normal. And I think that was helpful to Pat. I think it was good medicine for him."

And Andrew is right. Keeping my life active and normal was an elixir of life. If you are caring for someone with cancer, consider this: Perhaps the best thing you can do for that person is to keep his or her life as normal as possible. You may be tempted to pamper and hover over that person— and certainly there are times when a cancer patient needs a mother hen. But perhaps what that person needs most is an assurance that life goes on, and life can be more or less normal, even after a cancer diagnosis.

Step 4: Beware of Unscientific "Cures" and "Remedies"

After the press conference where I announced that I had cancer, my office was flooded with letters, e-mails, and phone calls from people urging me to replace chemotherapy with a certain diet, juice, powder, or pill. Many of these communications clearly came from hucksters who wanted to exploit my illness for their own gain. But the vast majority of this advice came from kindhearted people who wanted the best for me and who truly believed in the power of these "miracle cures."

I was amazed at how many people, seemingly with the best of intentions, urged me to reject medical science and stop going to the doctor. "Stay away from chemo!" they wrote. "It's poison!" Well, of course chemo is poison. That's how it works. It destroys the cancer cells. Yes, it's also hard on the good cells, but while it is killing the cancer cells, it's saving my life.

There are many so-called poisons that we need in order to live, from minerals like selenium (vital for cell function yet toxic in high doses) to certain vitamins (which can also be toxic in high doses). Even oxygen in sufficiently high concentrations can cause cell damage and death. So calling chemo a "poison" is meaningless. If medical science has shown that a "poison" can save the life of a cancer patient, then we need to stop calling it a "poison" and start calling it a "wonder drug."

People have urged me to follow the most bizarre diets imaginable. They've urged me to eat exotic leaves from the rain forests of South America, or extracts from berries harvested from a remote island in the South Pacific, or some strange secret-formula powder that you mix with water. These "cures" are all expensive—but, the sales pitch goes, what is it worth to you if it cures your cancer?

The people who offer these "cures" are relentless. They do not give up. I always tried to be gracious and kind, and to thank people for their concern. "Can we send you a sample?" they'd ask. "Yes, go ahead," I'd say. I always hoped that would put an end to it. But a few days later, they'd call back. "What did you think of our product? How do you feel? How many cases would you like to order?" It never ends. If you take their sample, they think they've got you on the hook, and they never stop trying to reel you in.

And I will admit to a very common human frailty: part of me wants to believe. When you have cancer, and someone tells you, "I will sell you the cure for cancer for just $399.99 plus postage and handling," something inside you asks, "What if it's true? What if it works? Are you sure you want to pass up the cure for cancer?" I'll be honest with you: I actually bought into a few of these phony "cures" before Ruth finally said to me, "Pat, what are you doing? You know those things don't work." We're not doing that. We'll buy our fruit and our juices at the grocery store. We're not going to order exotic foods and extracts from the ends of the earth to cure this cancer."

During one of my visits to Dr. Reynolds, I told him about all of these "cures" that people wanted me to try, and I asked him if there is any such thing as a "cancer diet." He assured me that no such thing exists.

"The closest thing to a 'cancer diet,'" he said, "is simply eating heart-healthy foods every day. As for those powders and juices people want to sell you, swindles like those have been going on since the old traveling medicine shows, and probably since the beginning of time. Pat, if I could dig worms out of the ground, grind them up, and feed them to you and make you well, I'd do it. Look out the window. See that tree? If I could take the leaves off that tree, grind them into powder, and stir it into a drink to make you well, I'd do it. If we could bottle it and sell it as the 'Incredible Magic Tree Cure-All,' we'd make millions. There are countless people out there who would reject the best treatment that medical science has to offer in favor of magic beans."

Dr. Reynolds reminded me that the "magic cure-all" approach had shortened the life of Apple founder Steve Jobs. In October 2003, Jobs—a Buddhist vegetarian—was diagnosed with a rare but curable cancer that was manifested in the form of neuroendocrine tumors of the pancreas. Though most forms of pancreatic cancer are far less curable, the cancer Jobs had was generally treated by surgically removing the tumor, along with a safe margin of tissue—and that treatment was usually successful.

But Jobs chose to pursue alternative treatment for nine months, from October 2003 through July 2004. By the time he finally agreed to undergo conventional medical cancer treatment, doctors had to remove his pancreas and duodenum. In 2009, doctors performed a liver transplant on Jobs. Experts say that it's unlikely that any of these more extreme procedures would have been necessary if Jobs had simply undergone commonsense cancer treatment immediately after he was diagnosed.[6]

Don't be embarrassed if you have fallen for a few of these "miracle cures" yourself. I'm right there with you. But thanks to Ruth and Dr. Reynolds, I quickly came to my senses. As I see it, I've got only one shot at beating cancer. If I blow my one and only chance at remission on some exotic powder or berry extract, I won't get another chance. So, when well-meaning folks or greedy hucksters try to get me offtrack, I simply say, "Thanks for your suggestion, but I'm going to do everything that Dr. Reynolds and Dr. Khaled have told me to do."

There's only one irreplaceable life per customer. Don't entrust yours to medicine show quacks and hucksters. Trust science and sound medical practice. Knowledge is power; fight cancer with real scientific knowledge and the latest medical advances.

Knowledge is power; fight cancer with real scientific knowledge and the latest medical advances.

We never know how much time we have left on this planet. All we know is that we have a responsibility to use the finite gift of time God has given us to serve him and do some good in this world. If you are battling cancer, one of the best ways to use the time you have left is to compete hard, to battle with all your might. There are no guarantees that the cancer won't take your life. That's okay, just keep battling hard. Fight bravely, fight wisely, fight strategically.

As long as you never surrender, you are never defeated.

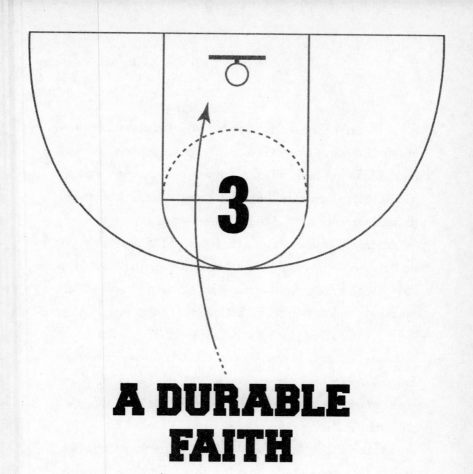

A DURABLE FAITH

Why me?

I admit it. After receiving the diagnosis of multiple myeloma, I wrestled with that question. *Why me? How could I have cancer? I've taken such good care of myself all my life precisely so I would never have to hear a doctor tell me, "Pat, you have cancer."*

For a brief time, I felt sorry for myself. I thought it was unfair. I wondered how God could allow it, especially after I had tried to live faithfully for him for so many years. I didn't stay in that place very long, but I would be dishonest if I didn't confess that I did think those thoughts.

Andrew says that it seemed to him that I "flipped a switch" on that kind of thinking almost instantly. Well, I assure you that it took a bit more than flipping a switch to get past my questions and, yes, some initial feelings of self-pity.

But soon after I began asking myself *Why me?*, another question occurred to me: *Why* not *me? Millions of people are diagnosed with cancer every year. Why should I be exempt? God won't allow me to go through anything I can't handle in his strength. He'll get me through this.*

I think the reason I was able to transition from *Why me?* to *Why* not *me?* was that I've spent the better part of a lifetime memorizing Scripture and trying to build biblical wisdom into my life. One of the first passages of Scripture that occurred to me after I learned I had cancer was 1 Peter 4:12–13: "Dear friends, do not be surprised at the fiery ordeal that has come on you to test you, as though something strange were happening to you. But rejoice inasmuch as you participate in the sufferings of Christ, so that you may be overjoyed when his glory is revealed."

Soon after those words from the New Testament came to my mind and altered my perspective, I encountered a quotation by Henry Blackaby, the noted speaker, Bible teacher, and author of *Experiencing God*. Speaking about God, Blackaby said, "He has the right to interrupt your life. He is Lord. When you accepted him as Lord, you gave Him the right to help Himself to your life anytime He wants." I have been hanging on to that statement throughout my cancer journey.

Another statement that I have treasured during my cancer battle is this quote from *A Sweet and Bitter Providence* by John Piper: "Life is not a straight line leading from one blessing to the next and then finally to heaven. Life is a winding and troubled road. Switchback after switchback. . . . God is for us in all these strange turns. God is not just showing up after the trouble and cleaning it up. He is plotting the course and managing the troubles with far-reaching purposes for our good and for the glory of Jesus Christ."[7]

"Since cancer, I feel like I have dreams rather than ambitions, visions rather than plans."

—Eve Ensler

Those words certainly describe the journey I've been on throughout my life. I have been incredibly blessed in so many ways, yet I have also experienced those windings and switchback turns that John Piper describes. Through it all, I have seen the guiding and providing hand of God—and his hand is with me in this cancer battle.

I committed my life to God when I was twenty-seven years old, and I have tried to live by faith and trust in him ever since. I've written about my faith and talked about my faith literally thousands of times over the years. Now comes the acid test. My crisis of cancer is going to reveal whether my faith actually means anything or not.

Every morning since this diagnosis, I have started the day with a choice to make: Will I be angry with God, accuse him of injustice, and pull away from him? Or will I continue trusting him and clinging to him?

Every single day, I've made the same decision: I'm clinging to him for dear life. I've crawled up into his lap and thrown my arms around his neck. I'm looking into his eyes and seeking his will. My faith has never been stronger.

I've never felt closer to God than I do at this moment.

"Thanking God Every Day"

The day Dr. Reynolds told me of my diagnosis, he also said that my strong faith in God would be a powerful weapon in my cancer battle. And he was right. My optimism and my focus on health and fitness have been strong allies in this battle, but my relationship with God has been far more encouraging, motivating, and comforting than all the other factors combined.

One Sunday morning, not long after I was diagnosed with cancer, I was greeted at church by Randall James, who is one of our pastors. He had just learned of my diagnosis and wanted to encourage me. In his deep-thicket drawl, he said, "Jesus could have prevented this, Pat, but he decided not to. God has a purpose for this trial in your life."

That is no empty platitude. In fact, that was a real turning-point statement in my cancer journey. I hadn't thought about that before. Yes, I knew that God could have prevented me from having cancer—but the idea that God actually had a purpose for my cancer was a new concept.

When Pastor James made that statement, he spoke from personal experience. Around First Baptist Church of Orlando, he's known as "The Cancer Pastor." In a moment, I'll let him tell you why. But first, let me tell you the advice he gave me.

"Pat," he said, "as you go through this cancer battle, I want you to recite the Lord's Prayer every day. But I want you to add a little twist to it. When you begin, say, 'Our Father, who art in heaven, hallowed *and healing* be thy name.' Don't forget to add those two words."

I took Pastor James's advice to heart, and I have been reciting the Lord's Prayer every day since, exactly as he encouraged me to do. It has helped me to focus on the mighty healing power of God in my life. With Pastor James's help, I've gradually been getting my faith legs under me, and I'm feeling more steady and stable in my trust relationship with God every day.

> I've gradually been getting my faith legs under me, and I'm feeling more steady and stable in my trust relationship with God every day.

Now, listen to Pastor James describe his own cancer journey. Before he begins, just two words of advice: brace yourself.

Pat Williams and I have been friends since around 1986. We go back to those early days when he was working hard to bring NBA basketball to Orlando. I have served as chief of staff to four Orlando mayors, and at that time I was working for Mayor Willard "Bill" Frederick. Pat took a huge risk, trying to build an NBA expansion franchise in a town that had no pro sports tradition. But the old adage proved true: "If you build it, they will come." They just don't make bold, risk-taking leaders like Pat Williams anymore—or like Mayor Bill Frederick. Both of them went way out on a limb and took big chances to make the dream of the Orlando Magic come true.

Since those days, Pat and I have been good friends—but we've become even closer since Pat was diagnosed with cancer. I've had the privilege of baptizing several of his grandchildren. I know exactly where he sits in church every

Sunday, and I often stop to chat with him and give him a hug after the service. I've also had the privilege of watching him battle cancer with courage and faith.

The Sunday morning Pat told me he'd been diagnosed with cancer, I shared with him one of my favorite sayings about adversity: "Nothing ever happens that is not Father-filtered." In other words, nothing happens to us that God the Father has not allowed in our lives for a reason. So I told Pat this, then I added, "Pat, let me tell you this: Jesus loves you more than your momma ever loves you." Now that's quite a statement for anyone who has experienced a mother's love. I love my momma so much, and she loved me, and I preached at her funeral—but the love of Jesus is even greater than a mother's love.

I told Pat, "If Jesus had wanted to stop this, he would have stopped this. But he's allowing you to go through this for a greater purpose. I believe God is going to use you as an example to others of God's power. In 2 Corinthians 1:3–4, Paul says, "Praise be to the God and Father of our Lord Jesus Christ, the Father of compassion and the God of all comfort, who comforts us in all our troubles, so that we can comfort those in any trouble with the comfort we ourselves receive from God."

I said, "That's what's going to happen, Pat. God is going to comfort you, and then he's going to use you to comfort others. I don't know whether that will take place through your speaking or through another book you'll write, but God is going to use you. Remember Romans 8:28, "And we know that in all things God works for the good of those who love him, who have been called according to his purpose." You may have to suffer through this cancer battle, Pat, but you won't have to suffer as much as Jesus suffered for you. He will never give you more than you can endure. He won't overload your plate.

Then I challenged Pat to memorize Isaiah 41:10: "So do not fear, for I am with you; do not be dismayed, for I am your God. I will strengthen you and help you; I will uphold you with my righteous right hand." That's a very special verse in my life. I was diagnosed with colon cancer in 1988, and my mother called me from North Carolina and said, "Son, I want you to memorize Isaiah 41:10. Then, before you go into surgery, you repeat that verse and see if it will bring you comfort." I memorized it, and I repeated it as I went into surgery, and I had no fear.

"We can look at our tattoos from
cancer treatment as awful reminders of
a ghastly time in our lives, or we can
use them as reminders of what
God brought us through."

—Shirley Corder

I told Pat, "If you memorize that verse, if you believe it's true, you have nothing to fear from the cancer. God will give you comfort and healing, and he'll use your journey through cancer to comfort others and bring glory to Jesus. Pat, as you go through this battle, God will bring cancer patients, myeloma patients, into your path. You'll be able to say to them, 'Look at me. I've gone through this illness. It's an incurable illness, but the Lord healed me and the same Lord who healed me can heal you, because he's the same Lord who created the heavens and the earth.' Pat, you've already spoken out boldly for the Lord, but he's fixin' to enlarge your influence. He could have given this important mission to someone else, but he has entrusted it to you, because he knows you will be faithful in adversity and you'll set an example to inspire others."

Those are just some of the things Pastor James told me in the very early days of my cancer battle. I've carried his advice with me through every hurdle and crisis along the way. I recited Isaiah 41:10 and the other Scripture passages he recommended to me again and again—and it's amazing how those words have lifted my spirits and taken away my fears.

Pastor James mentioned that he was first diagnosed with colon cancer in 1988. But you don't know the half of it. Again, listen as he tells you more about his experience with cancer:

I've had more than forty-five surgeries for cancer. That doesn't include open-heart surgery and some other surgeries that I've had. But I've had colon cancer, stomach cancer, lung cancer, throat cancer, skin cancer, a brain tumor, and I am being treated now for leukemia. So I've had at least one cancer surgery every year for the past quarter century.

After being treated for colon cancer, I was diagnosed with lung cancer in 1990. That came closer to killing me than anything else I've had. I got it from secondhand smoke. My dad was a heavy smoker—he died of lung cancer when he was fifty-nine. When I was little boy, I'd ride with him in the pickup all over North Carolina with the windows rolled up in the wintertime, breathing the smoke from his cigarettes.

I'm awaiting surgery now because we were in a critical car wreck, and four lumbar vertebrae were crushed. I've been receiving epidurals and cortisone for the pain for the past six weeks, but I haven't gotten any relief, so we're going to do surgery to relieve the pressure on my spine. My surgeon said that should take away my pain, so praise God!

One time, I felt short-winded, so I went to my cardiologist. He said, "Randall, you've got about an hour to live unless we can get you a blood transfusion." I said, "Doc, are you sure I've got that long?" He said, "Yeah, I think you have about an hour." I said, "That's just enough time." And I left the doctor's office, drove home, got my pajamas and my wife, and I was at the hospital, getting admitted, in less than forty-five minutes. That's when they took out my aortic valve and put in bovine tissue—I told the nurses that it was a cow's ear.

I decided a long time ago, I'm not going to let illness or pain steal my joy. I've learned to enjoy poor health, knowing that God is in control. Before every one of my surgeries, I recite Isaiah 41:10 as they prep me to put me to sleep. They always check my blood pressure and say, "Mr. James, do you know what we're going to do to you?" I say, "Yes, you're about to put me under and cut me open." They say, "But your blood pressure is a hundred twenty over eighty. Your pulse rate is perfectly normal. Most people going into surgery are scared."

"I decided a long time ago,
I'm not going to let illness or pain steal
my joy. I've learned to enjoy poor health,
knowing that God is in control."

—Randall James

But I'm never scared. Jesus is standing right here by me. He told me he would hold me by his right hand. So I'm not going to worry. Pat, you do the same thing. Trust God to walk through this journey with you and you'll see what he wants to do through your cancer.

I've been hospitalized twenty times in the past two years, and I've led eighteen nurses to faith in the Lord and I baptized one of them. I told the Lord, "Father, just give me the names of the nurses you want me to talk to, and I'll look them up and lead them to you. You don't have to keep sending me to the hospital." But God has seen fit to send me back to the hospital again and again. And since that's the way he has chosen to use me, and since I'm going in for back surgery again soon, I'm looking forward to it.

The Lord is my strength, and I've been through nothing compared to what Jesus has been through for me. We don't have to look very far to find somebody who is worse off than we are. When you see young men and women coming back from Iraq and Afghanistan with both legs missing or with burned faces and bodies, it changes your perspective.

I'm not going to complain about my life. I'm going to be a good sport about it. This too shall pass. I praise God that my life has been as good as it's been. I'm thanking God every single day.

And I thank God for Randall James, and for his impact on my life and my cancer journey.

The Proven Power of Prayer

Since my diagnosis became public, thousands of people have called or e-mailed me and told me they are praying for me—far too many to count. One call I received came from Bob Boone, a dear friend and a longtime major league catcher. He called me soon after the February 2011 press conference and said, "Pat, I want you to know that Sue and I will be praying for you."

Time passed. I went through months of chemotherapy, followed by a stem cell transplant. And I heard from Bob Boone again.

"Pat," he said, "how are you doing with this cancer fight?"

"I'm doing very well, Bob," I said.

"Is that the honest truth?"

"Bob, it's true. The doctors are very pleased with my progress. I'm on the right road and I'm very encouraged."

"Well, doggone it," he said. "I *thought* that prayer stuff works!"

Yes, it's true. That prayer stuff works. Countless people have been praying for me, the Lord has heard their prayers, and he's working in my life.

But *how* does that prayer stuff work?

Many doctors and researchers believe that prayer has about the same healing power as a sugar pill. They believe that if a patient knows he or she is being prayed for, there may be a "placebo effect"—the mysterious ability of the mind to help the body to heal itself. If you truly believe that prayer is as powerful as a wonder drug, they claim, then prayer will have healing power.

Doctors and researchers also know that the act of prayer is a good stress-reduction technique. Praying helps reduce stress, lower blood pressure, improve pain management, and promote gastrointestinal health.

Does prayer truly call upon God to release his healing power in our lives? You might be surprised to learn that the scientific evidence says yes.

But we have to wonder: Is there more to prayer than a placebo effect? Does prayer truly call upon God to release his healing power in our lives? You might be surprised to learn that the scientific evidence says yes.

In the 1980s, cardiologist Randolph Byrd conducted a double-blind experiment involving 393 randomly selected patients from a coronary care unit at San Francisco General Hospital. Patients were divided into prayed-for and not-prayed-for groups. Protestant and Catholic volunteers prayed to the Judeo-Christian God, asking for healing for people who were known to them only by a first name and diagnosis.

Each prayer volunteer prayed daily and specifically for a fast recovery and the prevention of complications. The experiment was controlled in such a way that the patients, doctors, and nurses did not know which patients were in the prayed-for group and which were not.

Researchers were surprised by the results. The study found that prayed-for patients were five times less likely to need antibiotics and three times less likely to develop fluid in the lungs than the not-prayed-for group. Almost every factor in patient recovery measured by Dr. Byrd's study appeared to be improved by prayer. Prayed-for patients experienced "fewer episodes of pneumonia, had fewer cardiac arrests, and were less frequently intubated and ventilated."[8]

The *Archives of Internal Medicine* published a parallel study eleven years later. In a controlled trial conducted by Dr. William H. Harris (a heart-disease researcher) at Saint Luke's Hospital in Kansas City, Missouri, doctors studied 990 patients with life-threatening heart conditions ranging from heart attacks to congestive heart failure. Of these patients, 466 were randomly assigned to a prayed-for group while 524 were assigned to a control group that was not prayed for.

Doctors and patients in the Kansas City trial were not even told that a clinical trial was being conducted, eliminating all possibility of bias. Seventy-five volunteers from various Protestant and Catholic churches prayed for the 466 prayer-group patients for twenty-eight days. At the end of that time, patients from both groups were evaluated according to thirty-five medical parameters. The prayed-for group scored 11 percent higher than the control group—a significant result. "This is a very well-designed study," said James Dalen, dean of the Arizona University School of Medicine and editor of the *Archives of Internal Medicine*. "If [prayer] was a medication, the conclusion would be that this medication helped."[9]

These studies show that prayer is a powerful force for healing—especially when combined with the best medical treatment available. Prayer is not a substitute for medical treatment, and we should never reject medical treatment in favor of prayer alone. We should also remember that prayer is not some sort of magic spell—it does not *guarantee* any particular outcome.

Prayer is the act of talking to God, listening to God, inviting his involvement in our healing and the healing of our loved ones. But God is sovereign, he is Lord, and we have to trust him and leave the final results in his hands.

"Cancer is such a wake-up call
to remind us how high the
cosmic stakes really are and how
short and brief and frail
life really is."

—Joni Eareckson Tada

As Henry Blackaby said, God has the right to interrupt our lives—and we need to be open to allowing God to use either our health or our illness to serve others and achieve his purposes in the world.

"Rest in the Hope"

This book is written not only to cancer patients, but to the loved ones of cancer patients—those who give care and support to those who are going through a cancer battle. After my diagnosis, my daughter Karyn, who is married and a singer-songwriter in Nashville, wrote a touching memoir of her emotions and faith journey after learning I had cancer.

I remember all the times when she was little, and she would climb up into my lap and throw her arms around my neck and hug me. Maybe that's why this statement I made at the February 2011 press conference seemed especially meaningful to Karyn: "I thought I was close to the Lord before, but now I'm sitting in his lap and hugging him around the neck." She placed that quote at the beginning of the memoir she wrote.

It's hard for me to read her words without tears in my eyes. But if you are caring for someone who is going through a cancer battle, and you want to know how to help that person through your faith and prayers, I think Karyn's message will help you. She wrote:

> The phone was ringing when I woke up one Friday morning in early February 2011. It was my brother-in-law Tracy. I answered and could tell immediately that something

was wrong. He asked if I had spoken to Dad. I hadn't. Tracy said, "You need to call him. He's talking to all the kids today."

I didn't ask Tracy what was wrong. I didn't want to hear it from anyone other than my dad. There are nineteen kids in my family, and there would be only one reason he was calling all of us on the same day—bad news. For the next hour I called every number I had for Dad, but I couldn't reach him. The more time that went by, the more anxious I felt. I sat on my couch and tried to calm down.

Finally, after what felt like an eternity, my phone rang. It was Dad. My voice shook as I answered the phone. "Hey, Dad, what's going on?"

His voice was calm, reassuring. "Karyn, I went in for a physical a few weeks ago, and I need to fill you in on what happened . . ."

My heart sank. He explained the diagnosis he'd received and the treatment he was about to embark on, including chemotherapy twice a week. After I heard the word *chemo*, I had a hard time processing what I was hearing. I heard Dad say something about a cancer called multiple myeloma, that it was in all of his bones except his skull, and I heard "no cure, no surgery" but "our goal is to get it into remission."

I thought, *Yeah, okay . . . remission . . . whatever. I'll process that later*. All I knew was that my dad had cancer. As we talked, I did my best to stay strong for him, but it was too late—my tears were already flowing.

We cried on the phone together until Dad finally said, "Karyn, God's going to use this. I'm absolutely convinced of that."

I have to be honest—in that moment my only thought was, *Let him use someone else!* But I did my best to console my dad, and he did his best to comfort me over the phone. In a matter of a few short minutes, my world had changed and my heart was shattered.

I hung up the phone and sat back down on my couch, stunned. I tried to breathe normally, but I felt the walls caving in around me. Finally, I let loose and screamed through my empty house, "Why, God, why?"

Not him, not my dad. Not the man I leaned on and needed so much in my life. Not the rock of our family, the man who has taught me everything I know about how to live my life, how to work hard, how to treat people with kindness, how to love the Lord. Do I have to sit here helpless and watch him die? No! It absolutely could not be happening.

I didn't know what to do next. I called my husband. I'm not the dramatic type, but today was different. "Come home!" I cried into the phone. "You have to come home right now." He dropped everything and ran.

I called my good friend and ever-faithful prayer warrior, Kim Boyce. I could barely speak, but I managed to say, "It's my dad—cancer." Kim instantly began praying. Because of Dad's position with the Orlando Magic, we couldn't talk to anyone else about his diagnosis until the story broke through the NBA.

I was scheduled to shoot my first music video a few days later. Looking at my red, puffy eyes in the mirror, I wondered how I'd get through the shoot. The video had been more than a year and a half in the making, and I wondered if I should reschedule it. Then I thought, *No, that's the last thing Dad would want.* I went through with my shoot, then went to Orlando to spend a few days with Dad and my family before the news broke publicly.

During the visit home, I walked downstairs one night and Dad was sitting up in bed. No one else was there, so I curled up next to him and we just sat in silence for a while. It's one of the things I have always appreciated about our relationship—our ability to just be together, not having to say anything.

"We wrote the song I'd been trying to write for almost a year. It was inspired by what my dad had said at his press conference: 'I thought I was close to the Lord before, but now I'm sitting in his lap and hugging him around the neck.'"

—My daughter Karyn

Finally, Dad said that the shock of it all was finally settling in for him. He said, "I've asked God repeatedly, 'Lord, why did you do this to me? I don't understand. I've been serving you, writing about you, speaking for you.' The only answer I've gotten seems to be, 'Urgency, urgency. You haven't been urgent enough. I needed to get your attention. I'm going to pull you through this, but you've got to tell people with a sense of urgency that they've got to move.'"

I thought, *Dad is the most passionate, energetic, urgent man I know. If he's not telling people about the Lord with enough urgency, then we're all in trouble!*

I went and got my computer and played him my new song, "Only You." It would become the title track of my debut album. He listened, then through tears he said, "That's it, Karyn, that's the message the world needs to hear. Nothing else will matter in the end except whether or not we knew the Lord."

People often ask me how I'm handling Dad's cancer battle. The truth is I was in shock for about a month after learning the news. I woke up every morning thinking it was a bad dream—then remembering it was all true. I couldn't get through a day without melting into tears. My body went through the motions of my life, but I wasn't really there. A friend equated the emotions I felt with wading through Jell-O, and I think that's an accurate description.

Dad has taken better care of himself than anyone I've ever known. So the words "my dad has cancer" simply wouldn't register. Yet it was true, and I couldn't change it.

After a few weeks had passed, I realized how exhausted I was from questioning God. I sat on my bed crying one night, and I asked my husband, "Will I ever feel normal again?" I realized I had to make a choice. I could wallow in these feelings forever—or I could lay them down and trust the Lord with my dad's life. It took a while, but I finally chose to trust God.

I had to stand alongside Dad and fight. Feeling sad and sorry for him wouldn't accomplish anything. Being mad at God wouldn't accomplish anything either. It hurt and I couldn't understand it, but I had to accept it and trust that God had a purpose for my dad's cancer. I've had to remind myself many times that God never promised that life would be easy—but he promised he'd be right by our side through it all.

I tried several times to write a song about this experience, but I couldn't. I finally decided to stop trying. If a song would be born, it would have to happen in God's time.

In December 2011, I sat down to write with Trey Heffinger and my husband, Brian White. I talked to them about my dad's illness and my feelings about it—and that day, we wrote the song I'd been trying to write for almost a year. It was inspired by what my dad had said at his press conference:

"I thought I was close to the Lord before, but now I'm sitting in his lap and hugging him around the neck." The song we wrote, "Rest in the Hope," became my first single to play on Christian radio. These are the words of that song:

There you were like always
Right in the middle of my lonely
Just when I thought there was no way
And I was the only one
You showed up and called my name
With a love that completely changed me
And now I know

   You are the truth that never changes
   You are the love that came to save us I am yours
   Even through all my fear and sorrow
   Facing a new unknown tomorrow I am sure
   That I'm gonna rest in the hope that I'm yours

I spent so much time looking for you
When you were here all along
Reaching for me to carry me through
Even when I would fall
You were waiting patiently
For me to find the faith to just believe
Oh and now I see

   You are the truth that never changes
   You are the love that came to save us I am yours

Even through all my fear and sorrow
Facing a new unknown tomorrow I am sure
That I'm gonna rest in the hope that I'm yours

Nothing can separate us from the love you gave us
Oh it's everlasting
Nothing can separate us from the love you gave us
Oh and now I know[10]

It's incredibly painful to learn that someone you love has an incurable disease. But as I've watched my dad go through his cancer battle, my attitude toward trials in our lives has changed. I'm learning so many lessons as I watch him go through this crisis.

"Nothing takes God by surprise,
not even cancer."

—Shirley Corder

Once, when I was in Orlando, Dad and I were driving together and he said, "I'm running a little late for my chemo. Do you want me to drop you off at home or do you want to come with me?" I decided I wanted to see what his "cancer life" was like, so I went with him.

At the treatment center, the lady at the front desk smiled when Dad walked in. "Hello, Mr. Williams!" she said. "How are you today?" Dad touched her arm and chatted with her by name. Later, when we reached the nurse's station, it was a partylike atmosphere when the nurses spotted Dad. They hugged him, and he addressed each one by her first name or even a funny nickname. I saw him spreading smiles and joy everywhere he went—that was so typical of Dad.

Going to Dad's chemo appointment reaffirmed for me that we all have a choice to make in the midst of cancer. We can choose to walk around spreading doom and gloom—or we can say, like Dad, "Well, it's not what I would choose, but this is my journey now, and I'm going to handle it with grace, fun, and faith in God."

One of the hardest lessons in life is knowing that God allows certain painful events for a reason. As Pastor James has said, "Nothing happens to us that isn't Father-filtered." God has allowed cancer into Dad's life, so he obviously has a reason for it. If one more person meets Jesus through his cancer diagnosis, then it was all worth it. That's the hope we rest in.

I recently had Dallas pastor and broadcaster Tony Evans as a guest on my radio show. As we chatted, Tony said something that really struck home: "Hope means it's better where you're going than where you've been." I immediately wrote those words down. That's exactly what hope means to me. I am absolutely confident that no matter what lies ahead of me in this cancer battle, it's better where I'm going than where I've been. If I am victorious over this cancer, I can look forward to more years of enjoyment with my wife, children, and grandchildren. If the cancer takes my life, I look forward to eternity with the Lord. Either way, I have a great hope, and I am resting in that hope.

The Gift of Cancer

For most of my life, I've lived by faith in God. I've talked about God and written about God, and now it's time to see if I truly live out what I say I believe. Ever since I first heard the words "multiple myeloma" from my doctor, I've been sitting in God's lap, seeking his will.

Soon after I was diagnosed, I encountered a great quotation from an anonymous author: "What may seem upside-down to us is right-side up to God." It's true. I don't want to have cancer. I wish I could make it go away. Yet I can see that God has a new adventure for me at this time in my life.

Throughout my career, I've given motivational speeches to corporations, organizations, sports teams, and church groups. My core message: "Believe! Have faith! Live courageously! Be bold! Be positive! Persevere!" I always thought I lived out that message and those values when I was a minor league baseball general manager, when I was an NBA general manager with such teams as the Chicago Bulls and the

Philadelphia 76ers, and when I worked with Jimmy Hewitt and other Orlando business and civic leaders to turn the Magic dream into a reality.

But I have never faced a challenge like this before. I have never faced an oppo-nent like cancer. I have never fought a battle in which my mortal existence was on the line. Even so, I'm thankful God allowed this to happen. My cancer battle has changed

I have never faced a challenge like this before. I have never faced an opponent like cancer. I have never fought a battle in which my mortal existence was on the line. Even so, I'm thankful God allowed this to happen.

my life. I've told God I want him to use me. I've told him I want him to make me bolder and to give me a greater sense of urgency in speaking out about what truly matters in life. I want to become a spokesman for cancer research and men's health—but above all, I want to become a spokesman for faith in the Lord Jesus Christ.

If you are not a person of faith, I would encourage you to settle things with God right away, right now. This cancer battle is a fight I would not want to go through without the Lord by my side. He promises he will never leave us nor forsake us. And that is the promise I cling to every day.

Every week, I receive phone calls and e-mails from myeloma patients and other cancer patients. Some are believ-ers, some are not. Whenever I hear from someone who is dealing with cancer, I always make it clear to that person how he or she can have a personal relationship with the Lord. Ruth once said to me, "I can't fathom how anyone could go through a cancer battle without a personal relationship with the Lord. I don't know how they do it." And I don't know either.

Knowing Jesus Christ is not a matter of going to the right church, performing the right rituals, or doing enough good deeds. Jesus himself said, "For God so loved the world that he gave his one and only Son, that whoever believes in him shall not perish but have eternal life" (John 3:16 NIV). There are no strings attached. It's simply a matter of accepting the free gift of salvation through believing in Jesus Christ.

The Bible also tells us, "For it is by grace you have been saved, through faith—and this is not from yourselves, it is the gift of God—not by works, so that no one can boast" (Ephesians 2:8–9). You can't earn salvation—but you can receive it as a free gift from God. How do you receive this free gift? Simply by asking him. Let me suggest a prayer you can pray right now:

Heavenly Father,

Thank you for loving me and having a plan for my life. I confess that I've sinned many times, but Lord, I'm sorry for my sins, and I want to live for you from now on. I invite Jesus into my life as my Lord and Savior. Thank you for hearing my prayer. Please seal this decision and help me to live the rest of my life for you.

Thank you. In Jesus's name. Amen.

I know there are some people reading this book who may not want to hear this right now. I hope you won't think I'm trying to "force my religion" on you. If you aren't interested in knowing Jesus Christ, I hope you and I can still be friends. Even though I don't know you, I care about you and I want you to know him. It's only because I know Jesus Christ as my Friend and Lord that I can view this cancer as a gift, not a burden, and a blessing, not a curse. And that's why I'm so eager to share this message with you.

I believe the Lord has called me to a ministry of speaking and writing about cancer, and I believe it is God himself who has opened this door in my life. In recent months, Florida Hospital has asked me to help raise funds for a multiple myeloma center at the hospital. I now serve on the board of the Multiple Myeloma Research Foundation, founded by Kathy Giusti. Before I was diagnosed with myeloma, I had never heard of the disease. Now I'm a spokesman for myeloma research. The Lord has called me to this cancer battle, and I have submitted to his call. I'm out there fund-raising and speaking and meeting people one-on-one, doing what I can to raise awareness and help end the scourge of cancer. Just a few short years ago, cancer wasn't even on my radar.

"She knew God was bigger than
a pathology report. So she prayed."

—K. Howard Joslin

God chose a new field of leadership for me that I would never have chosen for myself. I'm eager and excited to see the next great adventure he is sending me on. I don't want to miss anything God has planned for me. I'm staying on the path he puts me on, wherever it leads. And I know that a day will come when I'll look back—and I'll be grateful.

For years, I've felt that there was another chapter in my life that would cap my career in baseball and basketball, and my career as a speaker and author. I wasn't sure how it would play out. To be candid, this is not exactly the chapter I was hoping for. But it's certainly an interesting one, and it's playing out even as I write these words. Whatever my next role may be, I know God has spent my entire lifetime preparing me for it.

I'm ready.

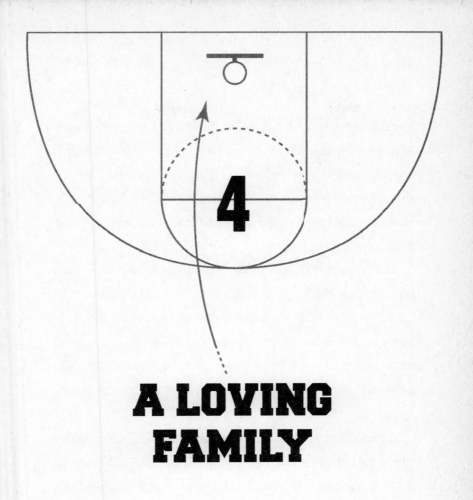

A LOVING
FAMILY

One of the hardest questions I faced after I was diagnosed was: how do I tell my nineteen children? As the father of four birth children, fourteen children by international adoption, and one by remarriage, all of whom are grown and have moved away, I found it a formidable task, both logistically and emotionally, to contact each one and explain the diagnosis.

We reached them all—and their reactions to the news were as individual as could be. Some were calm, some distraught, but all pledged to pray for me. After the press conference, they wore wristbands and T-shirts with THE MISSION IS REMISSION slogan printed on them. Their support has meant more to me than I can say.

Ruth has been my cheerleader. I don't know for sure, but I suspect she may have called the kids together and told them to be cheerleaders too. I can tell you this: My kids have never been gloomy around me. They've always been extremely positive. Maybe that's how they would naturally be in a situation like this—but I think I detect a touch of Ruth's wise, motherly coaching in all of this.

I remember when Ruth and I walked out of Dr. Reynolds's office, just after he had told me of the diagnosis. We stood on the sidewalk and looked at each other and shrugged our shoulders. Then Ruth said, "I'm with you, Pat. I love you and I'll support you through this."

And she has. She has always been exactly what I need through this cancer journey. She hasn't hovered over me or coddled me, because she knows that's not what I need or want. But she's always there when I need her to be there—an emotional and spiritual anchor, a friend, a prayer partner, and the one who took such excellent notes in Dr. Reynolds's office when I was in shock and unable to think straight.

Most important of all, Ruth has continued to live her life. She keeps her travel schedule and business appointments. I'm not saying she hasn't made sacrifices for me, because I know she has. But she hasn't set her life aside to be my nursemaid. If I was in my sickbed and Ruth was at my beck and call 24-7, constantly checking my temperature and cooling my fevered brow, we would both be miserable. But by keeping her life as normal as possible, she helps keep my life normal. And I need that.

The day Dr. Reynolds told me I had myeloma, he also told me that a major factor in my favor is the love and support of my family. It's true. Who could possibly have more love and support than a man with nineteen children and fourteen grandchildren? Maybe the reason I have so many children is because God knew I would need a lot of love and prayer support to get through this cancer battle.

This diagnosis has pulled our family together in a big way. . . . If you have the love of your family, whether you have one child or dozens, you have a great resource for healing and recovery.

"His Whole Family Is with Him"

Another great family resource in my life has been the love of my sisters, Carol and Ruthie. Sister Ruthie talked about the day I called her and told her that I had been diagnosed with multiple myeloma:

> When Pat called to tell me his diagnosis, he didn't even know what multiple myeloma was. I did. A friend of Mom's had multiple myeloma many years ago, back when there was almost nothing that could be done for it. So when Pat told me what he had, the only knowledge I had to draw on was the memory of this woman who had suffered terribly from myeloma back in the 1970s. I felt like I'd been hit by a truck. I was glad it was a phone call, so Pat couldn't see my eyes fill up with tears.
>
> At one point, Pat said, "Do you think I should tell everybody? I think maybe I won't."
>
> I said, "I think you should tell people, Pat, because I think the news will seep out around the edges. You don't want your family and friends to hear through some other source. You want them to hear it from you."
>
> He said, "Yes, you're right. My doctor gave me the same advice." Pat said his next call would be to our sister, Carol, who lives north of San Francisco. So we said good-bye. I had managed to hold it together throughout the call, but when I hung up the phone, I cried and cried.

Pat was the last person on the planet I would have expected to have this disease. He was the epitome of good health. He had never been hospitalized in his life—and he wouldn't even take aspirin. It wasn't right, it wasn't fair—but I had to accept it. I had to get over the sorrow so that I could be supportive to him.

It was winter when Pat called, the first Friday in February. We had a lot of snow that winter. I didn't know what to do to calm myself. I had no one to talk to. So I did the only thing I could think of: I put on my knee boots and went outside. I had a Leyland cypress tree in the yard, and it was bent over by snow and ice, stuck to the ground. I grabbed that tree and wrestled with it, trying to pull it upright. I just had to do something physical to work off this agony I felt.

Later, I thought of something more constructive to do. I don't have a computer, and I can't look things up on the Internet. So I went to the library and looked up myeloma in a cancer encyclopedia. The article was eight pages long, and the fact that my late husband was a physician helped me to make sense of some of the medical jargon. The article explained many of the recent advances in myeloma treatment. The information helped me to understand Pat's illness better, so I was less afraid.

Family has always been important to Pat. It was hard on Pat to go through the intensive chemo treatments prior to the stem cell transplant, because those treatments compromised his immune system and he had to be hospitalized and isolated from his children and grandchildren. One day, he called me from the hospital and said, "Ruthie, did you know how hard it is to sleep in the hospital?" Well, yes, anybody who's ever been in the hospital knows that the nurses are always coming in and waking you up to give you a sleeping pill or some such thing. But Pat had never been in the hospital before, so it was quite a revelation to him.

"When someone has cancer,
the whole family and everyone
who loves them does, too."

—Terri Clark

When you're going through an illness like cancer, little pleasures become very important to you. Pat had major chemo treatments in November and December 2011, before the stem cell transplant scheduled for February 2012. Because his immune system was compromised by the chemo, he was supposed to remain in isolation at home. But Pat wanted to go for a drive and see the Christmas lights and get a root beer float. So he talked Ruth into taking him out in the car—kind of a "jailbreak," because his doctors wanted him isolated. Ruth really wasn't happy that Pat was disobeying doctor's orders, but she went along with it because she knew how important these little pleasures were to him.

Pat called me from the car and said, "Ruthie, I called to tell you I escaped. I'm out in the car, cruising around Orlando, looking at the Christmas lights and drinking my root beer float." And he was just so happy to be out of the house and enjoying the Christmas season. I think it took him back to his boyhood, when Granny, our mother's mother, would come down from Pennsylvania. She loved to drive around Wilmington and look at all the Christmas lights. That was our Christmas entertainment when we were kids. Pat said, "Granny would be so happy if she could see all these lights!"

When you're going through a cancer battle, and it is so daunting, those little pleasures, those family memories, can cheer you up a lot. Even if you have to bend doctor's orders a little, those little family pleasures can be good medicine.

When I was recovering from the death of my husband and my mother, I began taking continuing education classes at the University of Delaware. One of the classes was a series of medical lectures. For one of these lectures, they brought in an orthopedic doctor, a bone doctor, to talk about multiple myeloma. It was very encouraging to attend his lecture, because he talked about the important advances that have been made in the treatment of myeloma. He explained why there is a much longer survival window for people with myeloma today than there was a few years ago.

When I told Pat I was attending a medical lecture to learn more about multiple myeloma, he was very touched that I had made that effort.

I have a coffee mug with the letter P on it, for Pat. I have my morning coffee from that mug, and it's a daily reminder of Pat. And I think of him often during the day. I pray for him, and the people here in our hometown of Wilmington all feel the same way about Pat. They often ask me how he's doing, and they tell me they are thinking of him and praying for him. When longtime friends call me, that's always the first question—"How's Pat?" And when I tell Pat this, he's always surprised that people have him on their minds. But they do. That's a comfort to him, and it's a comfort to me that friends and family and people we went to school with feel this strongly about him.

A cancer battle is a tough battle. But Pat is not going through this battle alone. His whole family is with him. I think that's a big factor in his healing.

My sister Ruthie is absolutely right. My family members are a great source of strength and encouragement for this battle, just as Dr. Reynolds said they'd be.

Kids and Grandkids

There are two principal ways that family members help strengthen a cancer patient to get through the cancer battle.

The first way is obvious: As family members, we support one another. We encourage one another, pray for one another, embrace one another, and express love to one another. That support flows from the family members to the cancer patient, lifting the patient's spirits and strengthening him for the daily challenge.

The second way is less obvious, but no less important: family members give us a reason to be strong. Because I have always focused on my health, because I have been a marathon runner, because I have always been active, energetic, and focused on my goals, some of my kids have seen me as a Rock of Gibraltar, practically invincible. Myeloma has made it abundantly clear that I am anything but invincible.

> **Family members give us a reason to be strong.**

Yet my children and grandchildren are still looking to me as a role model. They are watching me to see whether the "Rock of Gibraltar" crumbles under pressure or stands firm. Physically, I'm no longer a "rock." But I want to continue to be a rocklike example of faith and character to my family, especially my children and grandchildren. That responsibility to be a role model as I go through this battle actually strengthens me for the cancer battle.

My children, who are all grown, continue to go on about their busy lives, which is as it should be. But they continually call to check on my health, to tell me they're praying, and to ask about things that are going on in my life, such as the NBA draft. When this book is published, we will have fourteen grandkids. The oldest will be nine and the youngest will be about four months old. So it's a great spread of ages, and they bring me a lot of joy.

The only drawback to having a large family is that it was a huge logistical challenge to let all of my kids know that I had been diagnosed with cancer. I wanted to call each one personally, not just send out a mass e-mail. The problem in our family is that it doesn't take long, if you tell one person, for the news to spread through the circle. I felt terrible that Karyn found out from another family member that I had bad news to share—and that she then had to wait anxiously for a long time before learning what that news was.

With each phone call I made, I had to experience the same set of emotions again and again, both their emotions and mine. Again and again, when I said that I had cancer, I heard, "What? No!" And before long, many of my kids came rushing over to the house (eleven of them live in the Orlando area). I had to assure each one that I was doing well spiritually and emotionally, that I was in good medical hands, and that the doctors had given me encouraging prospects for remission.

One of the most delightful forms of support I've gotten from my family is a wall covered with bright, colorful drawings made by my grandchildren. Some of the drawings have inscriptions, such as "I'm praying for you, Poppers!"

Those pictures and those prayers are a great encouragement. I believe God is especially attentive to the prayers of children.

I'm also encouraged by my grandchildren because little children know what's important in life. They're focused on wonder, joy, fun, and enjoying life. My grandchildren never come to me and say, "Poppers, how is your myeloma?" They know I have an illness, but they are not focused on my illness. They ask me, "Can we go swimming today, Poppers? Will you take us out for pizza?" As far as they're concerned, I'm still their grandfather, living a normal life, doing grandfatherly things with my grandkids. That is very healing for me.

The Most Healing Act You Can Perform

When a family member enters a battle with cancer, the family will not remain the same. Cancer doesn't just invade one person. It invades the entire family, and the entire family must respond. Here are some of the responses that a cancer patient and the patient's family need to consider making:

Heal Family Wounds

Cancer forces us to realize what is important in our family relationships. It makes us conscious that our time together as a family is finite, and if any unhealed relational wounds exist between family members, it's time to come together and heal them. Cancer doesn't automatically bring people together, but it does confront us with a sense of urgency. Wise family members who understand the importance of love, compassion, and forgiveness will take the risks and make the effort to heal family rifts and divisions.

A person who is going through a cancer battle does not need the emotional upheaval of family fights, nor the emotional poison of bitterness and resentment. When you or someone else in the family is battling cancer, make the effort to heal family relationships. Healed relationships promote physical healing.

---

*"Like millions of others,
I have been plagued by the devastating
effects of cancer hitting not one, but
multiple members of my family."*

—Tom DeLonge

Make Faith a Family Priority

Your family may have wandered away from practicing a faith in God. You may have given up attending a house of worship. You may have neglected prayer and reading God's Word. It's time to come together as a family around a common core of faith.

You may say, "But I don't believe in God. Maybe I did once, but I don't anymore. If I go to church now, I would be a hypocrite." No, you wouldn't be a hypocrite. A hypocrite is someone who pretends to be something they're not. You don't have to pretend to be anything. You can simply go to church, be honest about your doubts or your unbelief, and say to the people in that church, "I simply can't bring myself to believe in God just yet. But our family needs help. We need to be surrounded by a healing community. We need to be accepted right where we are. We need to know we're not alone in this."

If you say those words in almost any church in the world, the believers in that church will accept you right where you are, surround you with love, help you, and go out of their way to meet your needs. Jesus taught his followers to love one another and to love others unconditionally, even those who believe differently than themselves. So if you and your family need a healing community right now, turn to the church. The church exists to reach out to people in need.

As a Family Member, Be a Reality Check for the Cancer Patient

And if you are the patient, draw upon the wisdom of your family members whenever you need a reality check. When people are diagnosed with cancer, they often get advice from friends and family. That advice is well-intentioned but often flawed. Patients sometimes make decisions for their own health care based on emotions, distorted thinking, or bad advice. As a family member, you need to help the patient think realistically about this disease and encourage him or her to seek the best possible information from his or her doctor.

Help the patient to write down questions to ask the doctor (it's important to have questions written down ahead of time, because it's easy during a visit to forget the most important questions we want to ask). Go with the patient if you can so that you can help ask questions, take notes, and listen to the answers. Encourage the patient to ask any question that is on his or her mind: Why are we doing this procedure? I read in a magazine about another procedure—why aren't we doing that? Why can't I have surgery for this cancer? What about holistic or homeopathic medicine? Help the patient sift through all the well-intentioned but often conflicting advice that he or she has been receiving.

Listen—and Be Honest

Take time to listen to the cancer patient, then respond honestly. But being honest doesn't mean you have to say everything you know. As a spouse or family member, you may have some knowledge or insight into the patient's treatment that the patient himself doesn't have. In some cases, the patient doesn't want to know all the details. His or her defense mechanisms are designed to help in coping with a frightening experience. If the patient doesn't want to know, you shouldn't feel obligated to tell him or her an unpleasant truth.

On the other hand, you must never lie. If the patient asks and clearly wants to know, then provide the information you have, simply and honestly. If the patient finds out you have lied to "protect" him or her from the truth, you will drive a wedge into your relationship. Knowledge can be healing power in the hands of a patient who can handle it. The patient needs to know that everything you say can be trusted. One of the worst feelings in the world is to be fighting for your life against a deadly disease and to feel that the people around you are keeping you in the dark.

Be aware of the protective mechanism known as denial. It's a stronger force than we generally realize. Denial often enables cancer patients to keep going when they are battling long odds. Denial isn't always a bad thing. It's closely allied with hope—the hope that everything is going to be okay. With today's advanced treatment technologies, that is

> Denial isn't always a bad thing. It's closely allied with hope—the hope that everything is going to be okay. With today's advanced treatment technologies, that is often a reasonable hope. So don't be too quick to take away a patient's denial.

often a reasonable hope. So don't be too quick to take away a patient's denial.

Dr. Reynolds told me, "I try to make sure I don't take anyone's hope away. I try to be honest, but not in a way that closes doors or destroys hope." If you want to help keep the patient alive, it's important to keep hope alive.

Stay Connected

When cancer strikes, it's not uncommon for some family members to pull away from the cancer patient. Some pull back because they don't know what to say. Others back away because of their fear of their own mortality. The whole subject of cancer is more than some people can face. Right when the cancer patient needs family relationships the most, people sometimes back away.

As a family member, you need to make a decision to stay connected with the cancer patient. Do you feel tongue-tied? Learn to ask questions, make conversation, hug, touch, and say, "I love you." Does the subject of cancer make you feel anxious and fearful? Well, everybody feels that way. Learn to act out of your compassion and courage, not your weakness and fear. The cancer patient needs you—he or she needs your love, your presence, and your strength.

Don't let your loved one feel abandoned. Stay connected. Demonstrate your love. Don't add to the hurt of your loved one; be part of the healing process.

As Family Members, Help the Cancer Patient to Live Normally

Ruth has walked through this cancer journey with me. She was there at Dr. Reynolds's office when he gave me the bad news. She went with me to several of my chemo sessions. She was there with me during the stem cell transplant sessions. But one of the most important things she did for me as I battled cancer was that she helped me to maintain a normal life.

Ruth understood—in fact, my whole family has understood—that I did not want to be treated like an invalid. I wanted to be able to go as far and do as much as my energy would allow. Ruth also observed when I was trying to do too much, and she would gently help to rein me in—not to limit me, but to help me conserve my energy so that I could live as normally as possible.

"When a person has cancer, the whole family really suffers with her."

—Ann Jillian

I don't like to go to the doctor. There have been several times when I allowed a simple cold to linger and turn into something bigger because I simply didn't want to be bothered with the doctor's visit. One time I ignored an infection in my hand for several days, and when I finally showed it to Dr. Khaled, he said, "Pat, this is serious. You need surgery on your hand." So he put me in the hospital, I underwent surgery, got out in a couple of days, and went on about my life.

As soon as Ruth finds out that I am letting a small health issue get bigger, she sends me to the doctor. Why? Because she knows that's the best way for me to live normally. If I don't want to end up spending weeks in bed like an invalid, I need to take care of these small health issues before they blow up into something big.

Sometimes, doctors and other healthcare professionals will tell a spouse or other caregivers, "Make sure the patient gets plenty of bed rest." Ruth knew there was no way to make Pat Williams get plenty of bed rest! I had places to go, speeches to give, books to write—and I couldn't do that from a sick bed.

While I was in the hospital, I was a model patient. I did everything my doctors told me to do—more or less. I got as much exercise as they would allow me, because that was important to my recovery. I was determined to get better.

After I got out of the hospital, I was on my own turf. I'll admit that I've done a few things that would make my doctors recoil in horror—if I told them. I'll admit that I took a few flights on germ-filled airplanes when my doctors wanted me to stay home. One time Ruth told me, "Pat Williams, if you get on that plane, I'm going to call Dr. Khaled!" I said, "Call him, call him!" as I kissed her good-bye and headed out the door.

The bottom line is that family members need to be sensitive to the tension between allowing a cancer patient to do too much and making the patient feel like an invalid. You have to find that delicate balance. You have to let the cancer patient live as normally as possible under the circumstances. At times that means letting that loved one get on a germy airplane. At other times, it means making that loved one go to the doctor before a cold becomes pneumonia.

On one occasion I went to give a speech at a hotel on Disney property in Orlando. It was at a time when my immune system was still compromised from the heavy chemo I had received. My doctors had okayed me to do the speech, as long as I wore a surgical mask to prevent me from inhaling airborne microbes. The doctors were always telling me, "Wear your mask!" Well, I wasn't going to do a speaking engagement wearing a surgical mask—it would be distracting, inhibiting, and would mask my features and muffle my voice. When you give a speech, your audience has to be able to hear you distinctly and see your facial expressions.

Dr. Reynolds knows that I bend his rules a bit. He once said, "The things Pat has done during his healing process would make us doctors cringe if we really knew. And we'd rather not know. But the end result is that Pat has been able to live an amazingly normal life, even with cancer, and it has worked out quite well for him."

While most of the chemo I received had only the mildest of side effects, there was one chemo treatment that caused me to lose my hair. So Ruth went with me to Joseph A. Banks and helped me pick out a couple of Indiana Jones–style hats, one brown and one black. I wore those hats to a few events, such as the 2012 NBA All-Star Weekend in Orlando, but I finally decided that if a cue-ball-smooth head was good enough for Michael Jordan, it was good enough for me—and I started going to events with my scalp au naturel.

Before I was diagnosed, my family often told me they wanted me to stop running marathons. They said that at age seventy, I was getting too old. So I asked them, "What's the worst that can happen?" They said, "You could drop dead." I said, "So what? I might drop dead running a marathon, doing what I love. That's not the worst way to go, is it?"

> As much as possible, if you are caring for a cancer patient, let that person live life on his or her own terms. A cancer diagnosis should not rob people of the life they want to live.

People ask Ruth, "How can you let Pat get on an airplane? How can you let him get up on a stage in a roomful of people who are coughing and sneezing and spreading all kinds of germs?" She says, "How can I stop him? If he drops dead onstage while giving a speech, he'll die the happiest man in the world. He'll die doing what he loves."

As much as possible, if you are caring for a cancer patient, let that person live life on his or her own terms. A cancer diagnosis should not rob people of the life they want to live.

When someone we love is sick, we want to protect them. That's understandable, and even admirable. But people often don't want to be protected. They don't want to be babied or coddled. They want to feel normal. They want to feel alive. So my best advice to you as a spouse, loved one, or caregiver is to let that person live as normally as humanly possible.

It may well be the most healing act you could perform.

Talking and Touching

Recently, when I was inducted into the Philadelphia Sports Hall of Fame, my sister Ruthie picked me up at the airport and drove me to the event. I was going through a time of acute neuropathy in my hands and feet, a sensation of both pain and numbness due to the anticancer drugs I had been taking. I guess she noticed that I was clenching and unclenching my hands, because she said to me, with emotion in her voice, "Just fight it, Pat. Fight it with all your might."

I'm grateful to have a cheerleader like Ruthie, urging me on through the biggest game of my life, urging me to fight on. My sister Ruthie is one of the many reasons I fight this battle. My sister Carol, who cheers me on from California, is another reason. My wife, Ruth, and my nineteen children are twenty more reasons.

The support of a loving family is a big motivator and a powerful source of strength for anyone who is in the throes of a cancer battle. If you are going through cancer right now, turn to your family for support. Lean on them, draw strength from them, nourish yourself with their love.

And if someone you love is fighting a cancer battle right now, join the battle and stand alongside that person. Say, "Fight it. Fight it with all your might. Don't give up. I'm here, I love you, I support you, I'm praying for you, I'm cheering you on."

Not long ago, I spoke at an event in Ocean City, Maryland, and Ruthie picked me up at the airport and drove me there. During the evening, we walked along the boardwalk and we talked about the days when we were growing up together—old times, good memories. Well, most of the memories were good, but I admit that I do have a few regrets.

For example, when we were growing up, I wasn't the most kind and thoughtful big brother in the world. I'm not saying I was particularly mean. I didn't go out of my way to be hurtful to my little sister. But I wasn't considerate of her feelings, either. I was a self-absorbed jock whose only thoughts were about sports. I look back on those days, and I savor the good times—but I also wince at the way I sometimes treated Ruthie.

As we walked along the boardwalk, talking and remembering the good times, I thought about all the love and support Ruthie had shown me over the years—and especially since my diagnosis. My heart was full to bursting with love for my kid sister. If only there were words to express how I felt at that moment.

"If you have a friend or
family member with breast cancer,
try not to look at her with 'sad eyes.'
Treat her like you always did;
just show a little extra love."

—Hoda Kotb

I haven't always been a touchy-feely, emotionally demonstrative person. But I have learned a lot in recent years about becoming more emotionally open and approachable. I've learned from my sisters, Ruthie and Carol, my wife, Ruth, my children, and other loved ones. I've also learned a lot from this cancer, because it has taught me about the urgency and importance of showing the ones you love how you truly feel—before it's too late.

So as we walked along the boardwalk, I reached out and took my sister's hand—a gesture that undoubtedly came as a jaw-dropping surprise to her. While the waves crashed on the shore below and the seagulls circled above us, we talked, laughed, reminisced—we were *family*. Walking hand in hand with my sister, I felt young again, and strong enough to conquer anything—

Including cancer.

If you have the support of a loving family, you have a reason to fight and a reason to live. You have the power to take on the world.

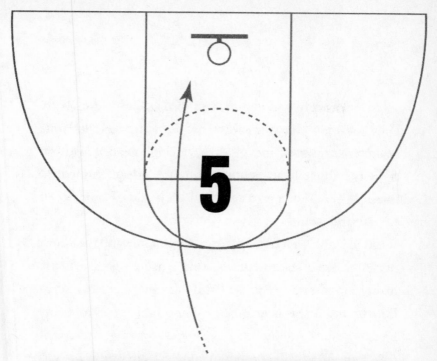

CARING FRIENDS

Shortly after I was diagnosed, and before I had made the public announcement, I was at the arena for a Magic home game. I found Magic co-owner Rich DeVos in one of the dining areas with his wife, Helen. I got Rich's attention, and he and Helen came over. "Hi, Pat," he said. "What's up?"

"Rich," I said, "I've just been to the doctor and I've been diagnosed with multiple myeloma—cancer of the plasma cells."

I saw concern and compassion well up in his eyes. "Oh, Pat," he said. "I'm so sorry." Rich has been through numerous health crises himself, including cancer and a heart transplant, so he is intimately acquainted with life-and-death medical issues. We sat down on a sofa, and Rich said, "Pat, we need to pray about this."

Rich and Helen put their arms around me and they both prayed for me. The realization that I had a deadly disease in my blood and bones was still very new to me, and as they prayed, I was overcome by emotion. I reached for my handkerchief and dabbed at my eyes. I was grateful that this man who had been my mentor, friend, brother in the Lord, and boss—while also being one of the wealthiest, most influential men in America—was at my side, lifting me up in prayer to God.

Sometime later, more than two years after my diagnosis, I talked to Rich again, and he said, "Helen and I pray for you almost every day." I was touched by the fact that he still continued to pray for me.

I also noticed that he said "*almost* every day." Many people will use empty platitudes and phrases like, "I'm praying for you," or even, "I pray for you every day." And sometimes you wonder, *Do they?* But Rich is a man of godly integrity, and he has many people on his prayer list—but he doesn't make empty claims. He won't say he prays for you every single day if it's really five times a week.

Just to have a place on Rich's prayer list is a rare privilege, and I'm sure his prayers are having an enormous impact on my life.

My Point Man

The day Dr. Reynolds told me my diagnosis, he also said that a major factor in my favor was the support and care of so many people in the Orlando Magic organization, the team I helped to found, beginning in 1986. I have received cards, notes, e-mails, calls, visits, and face-to-face words of encouragement from people at every level of the organization. Many of them have shared with me their own stories of battling and beating cancer.

"Having cancer gave me membership in an elite club I'd rather not belong to."

—Gilda Radner

One of the caring friends who has meant so much to me in my cancer battle is my assistant, Andrew Herdliska. He kept me organized, focused, and scheduled—and in this way, he kept my professional life normal. He didn't lighten up on me because I had cancer. He knew I didn't want to be treated like a "victim" of a disease. I wanted to keep my life moving forward. So Andrew would always tell me, "Okay, Pat, it's time to get ready for the next speech. I'm sending you to Houston tomorrow, and when you get back, you'll have a speech here in Orlando, then you're off to Philadelphia. Rest when you can."

I'm afraid that when I gave the news of my diagnosis to Andrew and the rest of my friends on the Magic staff, I didn't fully understand how they would be affected. Andrew recently talked about that day:

> When the diagnosis came down, Pat told the staff, "I had a doctor's appointment, and my doctor told me I have multiple myeloma." That's all he said. He didn't explain it at all. Then he went to his office and started his day.
>
> All of us in the office just sort of looked at one another, not knowing what to say. So I went to my computer and Googled "multiple myeloma," read for a couple of minutes—and didn't like what I read. I went to Pat's office and said, "That's cancer."
>
> Pat said, "Yeah, I know." He was so matter-of-fact about it that I couldn't tell if he was in shock, or if he simply refused to let it get to him. Was he merely being stoic for the sake of the staff? How is a person supposed to respond when they know they have cancer? I wasn't sure—but you don't expect a person to be matter-of-fact about something as serious, deadly, and incurable as myeloma.

I knew that we had to immediately begin dealing with issues surrounding the cancer. Who already knows about the diagnosis? Who should we tell? How do we make sure that only accurate information goes out, not rumor and hearsay? If Pat has already told his family, then it's going to be impossible to keep it a secret. With so many children and friends, Pat wasn't going to keep this story out of the media.

Andrew was thinking about all the details and potential problems that I was unable to focus on—and that was exactly what I needed. He became my point man in dealing with the logistics of the announcement. He was my liaison with the Orlando Magic press team during preparations for the press conference in February 2011. Andrew helped arrange for a local reporter to come to my house and interview me about the cancer battle for a newspaper piece that would appear after the press conference. He also arranged for printing up the T-shirts with the slogan THE MISSION IS REMISSION that my family and I wore at the press conference.

"How is a person supposed to respond when they know they have cancer?"

—My assistant, Andrew Herdliska

Andrew is much more than my assistant at the Magic. He's my friend—and he went above and beyond the call of duty in helping to keep my life normal as I continued to represent the Magic while fighting a life-and-death battle against cancer.

The Best Cancer Care May Be in Your Own Backyard

Another great friend and ally in my cancer battle has been the Orlando Magic's human resources director, Audra Hollifield. It was Audra, of course, who sent me for an executive physical at Florida Hospital's Celebration Health Assessment Center—and in doing so probably saved my life. If not for her, I might not be writing these words today. Audra recently talked about the day she learned about my diagnosis.

In late January 2011, I flew back to Orlando from Jamaica. After the plane landed, I checked my phone and had a voicemail from Pat. He said, "Aud, it's Pat. There's something serious about my health. We need to talk as soon as possible."

My heart sank. I immediately called him, and he said, "I went for this physical, and I was diagnosed with multiple myeloma." At that point, I didn't know what that meant. I don't think Pat knew much about myeloma either at that point.

I said, "Where are you?"

He said, "I'm at work."

Well, of course, he was at work. It was past closing time—where else would Pat be? I suggested we go to dinner along with Andrew. So the three of us met at a restaurant, and Pat told me about his diagnosis over dinner.

As Pat explained the situation, I found myself feeling hopeless. As always, Pat framed the situation as positively as he could—but I was simply not able to think positively. All I could think was, *How is Pat ever going to overcome this? It's incurable! It's cancer!* I kept thinking the worst.

Later, when I prepared to break the news to my staff, I thought, *What am I going to tell them?* I was not at a good place. By that time, I had read on the Internet about multiple myeloma, and I had a better sense of what this disease is and the treatment advances that have been made. I also knew that having a positive mental attitude can be a big factor in surviving long-term with myeloma. I wanted to believe the best for my friend Pat, yet I couldn't help thinking the worst.

I would watch Pat go through this day, and he was just so positive and upbeat. If it was anyone else, you might wonder, *Is he out of touch with reality? Doesn't he know how serious this is?* But it made me realize that Pat understood something that most of us miss: You have to be positive in a situation like this. Pat was only living what he had always preached. I had been around him for years, listening to him talk about staying focused on the positive, but a lot of people preach that. Pat really lives it. His cancer crisis revealed his true attitude about life—and his attitude today is the same attitude he's always had: stay positive, have faith, don't worry, take life day by day, and give each day everything you've got.

But here's the amazing thing: The more I learned about Pat's medical situation and about multiple myeloma, the more I realized that Pat really did have reason for optimism. His doctors had an excellent success rate in treating this form of cancer.

"Cancer affects all of us, whether you're a daughter, mother, sister, friend, coworker, doctor, patient."

—Jennifer Aniston

After Pat announced his diagnosis at the press conference, he got calls from a number of well-connected people who offered to help him get to some of the most eminent doctors and elite cancer clinics around the country. If Pat had taken any of those offers, he might have been flying all over the country to this or that cancer clinic, living in hotels, and turning his family's life upside down in order to get Cadillac-style medical treatment.

But Pat didn't go that route. I don't think he even consid-
ered it. He went to Florida Hospital, to his own doctors, Dr.
Reynolds and Dr. Khaled. He received most of his medical
care at offices within a fifteen-minute drive from home. And
they did an amazing job taking care of him.

Many people have asked me about Pat's health care.
They ask if he went to the M. D. Anderson Center in Houston, Sloan-Kettering in New York, or the Mayo Clinic in
Minnesota. I say, "No, he gets top-notch care right here in
Orlando." I think one of the lessons of Pat's cancer journey
is that you need to have faith in the medical community
around you. Pat says, "These are the doctors God brought
to me, and they're the doctors I'm going to put my trust in."

And Pat's doing great. He has plenty of air travel and
hotel rooms in his life. He doesn't need to complicate his life
further. So he gets all his cancer treatment a short drive from
home. Most of us have excellent doctors right in our own
backyards. This doesn't mean we shouldn't do the research.
We should. We should make sure that our doctors come
highly recommended. But if you're diagnosed with cancer,
you shouldn't automatically assume you have to travel a great
distance to find the best care.

Audra is right. I felt my life was in the very best hands
right here in Orlando. I remember well one call I received
from a longtime friend who offered to help me get into

an elite facility in New York or Boston. I was touched and amazed at his kindness, and I thanked him profusely and said I would think about it. I didn't really want to go that far from home to get treatment, but just to be safe, I mentioned my friend's offer to Dr. Reynolds. I said, "A friend has encouraged me to go to one of the prestigious clinics in the Northeast. What do you think?"

"Well," Dr. Reynolds said, "let me put it this way: I just got off the phone with the top myeloma doctor at the Dana-Farber/Harvard Cancer Center in Boston. I left a message and she called me back within two minutes. I told her what my plan was for you. She agreed that it was a hundred percent the right thing to do. Pat, we in the myeloma community are all in touch with one another. They're not doing anything at Dana-Farber that we're not doing here. From my perspective, there's only one reason you wouldn't want to have your treatment here, and that's if you're not satisfied with the nursing care."

I laughed. "The nurses here are like angels," I said. "They're the most kind, self-sacrificing people I've ever met—I wouldn't want to be anywhere else."

So I never gave it another thought after that. Why travel far from home and go to a strange city at thousands of dollars of extra expense when the care I need is right down the street? I can get more work done and spend more time with my family, and I can eliminate a lot of stress and conserve my energy—and all of those factors can be very important allies in my cancer battle.

I'm grateful to a number of friends around the country who offered to help me get the best care available. I'll never forget their kindness. But I'm grateful that the best care imaginable was available right in our own neighborhood. If you are considering where you should go for your cancer care, or where your loved one should go, I urge you to do your research. Get references and referrals. Gather all the insight and information you can. You may decide to go to a cancer clinic in some other part of the country. That's fine. But make sure you at least look into the cancer care options that are right in your own backyard.

> Do your research. Get references and referrals. Gather all the insight and information you can. You may decide to go to a cancer clinic in some other part of the country. That's fine. But make sure you at least look into the cancer care options that are right in your own backyard.

What a Friend Can Do and Say

Sometimes friends can fill a role in a cancer patient's life that family members can't fill. One time I was working late at the office, driving myself to get just a little bit more work done before heading home. I felt depleted after a round of chemotherapy, and for days I had been racked with a hacking cough. Ruth had been encouraging me to come home early and get more rest—but you know how it is. If your wife says, "You need to get more rest," you just say, "I'm fine; I'll tough it out. I really need to get this work done." So there I was, working and coughing—and I had gotten so used to the cough that I hardly even noticed it.

But Audra could hear it down the hall. She came to my office and said, "Pat, it's seven-thirty at night, your cough sounds terrible, and you need rest. What are you doing?"

"Well, I'm working on—"

"Whatever it is will still be here tomorrow. Pat, you need to take care of your health. Pack up your stuff. Get out, go home. There's no need for you to be at work this late."

And when she put it that way, I realized she was right. My wife had tried to tell me the same thing—and I should have listened to her. But somehow, the same advice sounded different coming from the human resources director, who also happened to be a good friend.

If you are a cancer patient, listen to your friends when they give you good advice. And if you are a friend of a cancer patient, don't hesitate to say what needs to be said. That person may listen to you when he or she won't listen to anyone else. Let me suggest to you a number of specific things you can do and say to be a supportive friend to a cancer patient:

1. *Be present.* This sounds too simple, but it's absolutely
   true. Cancer patients need you to just be there.
   Many patients feel ignored or abandoned. Friends
   stop calling because they don't know what to say, or
   because the idea of cancer makes them anxious and
   uncomfortable. Don't let this happen to your friend.
   Be present, be available. Call or e-mail. Give hugs or
   a touch on the hand. Don't feel you have to talk or
   offer advice or platitudes.

   You may say to yourself, "What if I can't find
   the right words?" That's just it—there are no right
   words. There's nothing you can say to make cancer
   better. You may say to yourself, *What if I get tongue-
   tied?* Don't worry about it. No one expects you to
   give a speech. Just be a friend. It's not your job to
   cure, but to care.

   It's okay to simply be present without saying
   a word. If your friend wants to talk, listen. If your
   friend asks, "Why?" don't feel you have to come up
   with an answer. Your friend doesn't expect you to fix
   things that can't be fixed. You can't make the cancer
   go away, but you can help your friend feel loved—
   and that will help him or her feel a lot less lonely
   and scared.

2. *Don't feel compelled to talk about cancer.* Don't avoid
   the subject, don't change the subject, but don't feel

you need to make cancer the topic of conversation. Be sensitive to your friend's thoughts and emotions. If he or she seems to want to talk about cancer, go with that. Your friend may want to talk through issues and feelings about the illness. Don't avoid any subject simply because it makes you feel anxious or uncomfortable.

"When I was diagnosed I didn't know how epidemic cancer was. You find out that everybody you know is touched by this disease."

—Laura Ziskin

If your friend doesn't want to talk about cancer, find something else to talk about, or just be silently present. Sometimes talking about memories, plans, kids, and events can help your friend feel more normal. Cancer patients want to feel that life is continuing on. Sometimes other subjects are a great distraction from cancer.

Above all, be a good listener. Talk about what your friend wants to talk about.

3. *Send supportive cards and notes.* E-mails are okay, but handwritten messages are even better. Write messages of encouragement, stories, remembrances, Scripture verses, and words of love and affection. Handwritten cards and notes become especially meaningful to cancer patients because handwriting is particularly personal, and these messages can be read again and again whenever encouragement is needed.

   People who are going through surgery or chemotherapy often don't have a lot of energy for a phone call, and unless you have gone through such treatments for cancer yourself, you may not realize how much energy it takes for a patient to talk on the phone. But handwritten cards pack a lot of uplifting emotional power while costing the patient very little energy to read. If you want to encourage your friends in a very big way, send a little note or card.

4. *Be sensitive to the patient's needs during hospital visits.* Check with family members or medical staff to see if your friend tires easily. Make sure you don't overstay your welcome or your friend's limited energy quotient. Some cancer patients hesitate to say, "I'm really tired now; I feel a nap coming on." Make sure you are sensitive to your friend's feelings

and strength level. If in doubt, ask, "Are you tired? I can come back tomorrow."

5. *Plan an outing.* If your friend is well enough, make plans to go out to lunch, just the two of you, or go boating or golfing, take in a concert or a play, or go for a drive in the country. An outing helps your friend feel normal, alive, and engaged in life. Such trips give cancer patients something to look forward to, and are always therapeutic.

6. *Offer to help your friend.* And when you offer, mean it. Many people say, "If there's anything I can do, just call me." Some people mean it, some don't. But most cancer patients are unlikely to ask for help. They often think, *I know she said I should call if I need anything, but I hate to be a bother.* Even if you invite people to call you, they almost certainly won't call.

   How, then, do you offer help to your friend? You do so by making a specific offer. Instead of saying, "Call me," say, "Can I drive you to your appointment? Can I make some phone calls for you? Can I do your grocery shopping or banking for you? Can I take your kids on an outing so you can rest?" Instead of asking, you may simply want to volunteer: "I'd be happy to do the vacuuming or mow your lawn. I brought my tools over, and I'm going to fix that broken screen door. I'm going to go pick up something for dinner—what would you like?"

In some cases, instead of asking or volunteering, you may simply want to pitch in and do something for your friend. Wash the car, bring over dinner, or take out the garbage. Don't ask—just do it. Offering practical help to your friend is a great way to show support and provide encouragement.

7. *Be germ-conscious.* Cancer patients frequently have compromised immune systems due to chemotherapy or other issues. If you have sniffles or a scratchy throat, stay away. Let your friend know that you don't want to pass along a possible cold or flu, but you'll visit as soon as you're sure you're not contagious. Your friend will appreciate your thoughtfulness.

8. *Donate leave time to your friend at work.* Many companies allow employees to donate unused vacation days or sick days to coworkers who are going through a cancer battle. Donating vacation time or sick leave to your friend is a meaningful gesture of caring. You can also donate blood or donate hair for wigs (to learn more, search online for Pantene Beautiful Lengths Program). Shaving your scalp is a great way to demonstrate solidarity with a chemo patient.

9. *Know what NOT to say.* Avoid saying anything
    hurtful or insensitive. Don't offer a cancer patient
    empty platitudes or false reassurance. For example,
    don't ever say, "Everything will be okay."
    A cancer patient knows that no one can make
    such guarantees. Don't say, "I know what you're going
    through," unless you are a cancer survivor yourself,
    and you really know what your friend is going
    through.

    Don't talk about people you know who have died
    from cancer. Don't talk about death unless your
    friend wants to talk about it. Don't take away your
    friend's hope. Cancer patients are well aware that
    death is a possible outcome, but the good news is
    that the majority of people who are diagnosed with
    cancer survive for five years or more. Encourage
    your friend to maintain optimism. Motivate your
    friend to fight hard. Inspire your friend to
    overcome adversity.

> Don't offer a cancer patient empty platitudes or false reassurance. For example, don't ever say, "Everything will be okay." A cancer patient knows that no one can make such guarantees. Don't say, "I know what you're going through," unless you are a cancer survivor yourself, and you really know what your friend is going through.

Don't urge a cancer patient to try alternative, nonmedical "cancer cures." Don't undermine your friend's trust in his or her doctors. Don't encourage your friend to abandon modern medicine.

Avoid saying, "I told you so." It's not helpful to tell a cancer patient, "I warned you to stop smoking," or, "I told you not to eat red meat." If you are not going to say something encouraging to your friend, then just sit quietly or go away. Words of accusation or condemnation can only cause harm to your friend's healing and recovery process. If it's not positive, if it's not helpful, don't say it.

Don't tell your friend how he or she should feel. For example, you should not say, "Don't be sad." While we can always choose our attitude, we can't always choose our emotions. Someone who has been diagnosed with cancer has every right to be sad, tired, worried, or scared. You may not be comfortable with a cancer patient's emotions, but so what? Your friend is fighting for his or her life. Accept and acknowledge your friend's feelings. Offer comfort, affirmation, and presence—not guilt or condemnation.

> *"When they tell you that you
> have cancer, you panic."*
>
> —Sofia Vergara

10. *Know what you SHOULD say.* There are a number
of ways you can express empathy and compassion
that your friend will find comforting. Here are
some things you can say that can be helpful and
encouraging: "I'm so sorry you're going through
this." "I know this is hard, but I'm with you." "I'm
thinking of you and praying for you."

If your friend asks, "Why me? What did I do to
deserve this?" you might respond with a variation on
the words Dr. Wilson said to me after he received
the report on my blood work: "Why do bad things
happen to all the good people?" Tell your friend,
"Cancer is an illness, not a punishment. Cancer
strikes saints and sinners, rich and poor, young and
old. You didn't do anything to deserve this, but I'm
going to be here with you all the way through it."

You don't have to answer the "why" question.
There is no answer to the "why" question this
side of eternity. But there are other questions
swirling in a cancer patient's mind that you *can*

answer—questions like, "Will my friends turn their backs on me? Will I be alone? Will I be abandoned?"

Your answer to those questions will be, "I'll listen to you, help you, comfort you, and calm your fears. I'm not going anywhere; I'm staying right here. I'm with you, and I won't abandon you. I'm your friend."

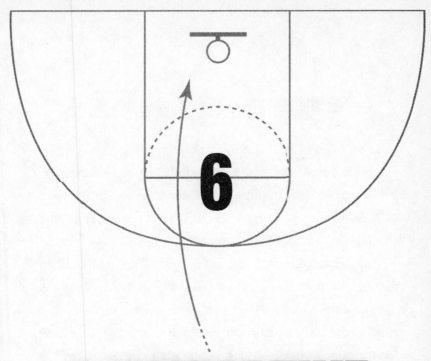

A SUPPORTIVE
COMMUNITY

The day Dr. Reynolds told me I had cancer, he predicted that a major factor in my healing would be the support of the Orlando community. He knew I had enjoyed a close and rewarding relationship with the Central Florida community ever since my early efforts to bring an NBA franchise to Orlando. "Pat," he said, "you're going to hear from this community. The people are going to rally around you in a mighty way."

He couldn't have been more correct.

Immediately after the February 2011 press conference, I was overwhelmed with e-mails, cards, letters, and phone calls. It was an amazing outpouring of support from the community. I received best wishes from all across Central Florida and all around the world. I heard from people I had met at different stages of my life, and I heard from many complete strangers. All were part of my community. At some time in the past, I'd had some influence or impact on their lives, and now they were contacting me to influence my life and support me in my time of need.

When I would go to the arena for home games, people would come up to me and say, "How are you doing, Pat? What's the latest news? We're pulling for you. We're praying for you." I can't tell you how much those words lifted my spirits.

Your community is your sphere of influence. Your community might be as small as your immediate neighborhood or as large as the whole world. Because of my travels, books, and media appearances, I have had the privilege of being part of a very large community. For years I've invested in this vast community of basketball fans, listeners, readers, and viewers, and now the investment is paying dividends, as countless members of this community express their support at this difficult time in my life.

How have you invested in your community? You have probably invested more than you realize. You've probably donated time serving others in your church. You may have volunteered to help your neighbors repair a fence, or you've given time to read to the children at the local kindergarten. You may have tutored in an after-school learning program. You may have simply been a good neighbor to the friends who live on either side of you and across the street.

If you have invested in your community, your community will repay you with dividends in your time of need. When you have needs, people you haven't seen in years will be there for you. You'll receive cards, e-mails, and phone calls. You'll be overwhelmed by good wishes and offers of prayer.

> If you have invested in your community, your community will repay you with dividends in your time of need.

And as it was for me, the support you receive from your community will be a big factor in your cancer battle and recovery.

A Christmas Diagnosis

Many if not most of us have a holiday tradition of watching Frank Capra's *It's a Wonderful Life*. We think it's a charming story about George Bailey (played by Jimmy Stewart), a man on the brink of suicide who is visited by a Christmas angel, Clarence (played by Henry Travers). Clarence reveals to him all of the many lives he has touched over his lifetime. The final scene leaves us with a warm, sentimental feeling for George and his family.

But we often fail to grasp the underlying message of the film—that *you* are George Bailey and *I* am George Bailey. We all touch so many lives, day after day, without even realizing the impact and influence we have. If a Christmas angel could come to us and reveal all the lives we have touched over the years, we would truly be astonished. My cancer diagnosis has been a lot like George Bailey's Christmas angel. When people heard that I had a life-threatening illness, they stepped out of the past and back into my life to tell me how I had influenced their lives.

Not long ago, I took part in a national sports forum in Orlando. During the program, a man stood up, looked at me, and said to the audience, "There is a man in this room tonight who had a huge impact on my life. I'm not sure he would remember me, but I want him to know how much I appreciate what he did for me. In the late 1990s, I was looking for a career in professional sports, but I was having no luck. Then I stumbled across a book he had written. He had his e-mail address printed in the back of the book, so I wrote to him. He wrote back, gave me his phone number, and told me to call him. We had a conversation I'll never forget. I was on the verge of quitting, and he inspired me to keep going. I soon found a job, and I've been working in professional sports ever since."

I don't know who that man was. I don't remember the conversation. But when he stood in front of that audience and publicly thanked me for having inspired him to keep going, he inspired me in a big way. He impacted my life and my spirit. I suspect his words may have even fired up my immune system and revved up my body's healing powers. At that moment, I knew how George Bailey felt at the end of the movie when his friends toasted him as "the richest man in town."

Around that same time, I also learned that two NBA players, Kevin Durant of the Oklahoma City Thunder and Mickaël Piétrus of the Toronto Raptors, both tweeted their best wishes for my recovery on their Twitter accounts. I knew Mickaël from the time he spent with the Orlando Magic, but I had never met Kevin before. It was a blessing to receive best wishes from these two NBA players.

"I feel I lost my
innocence to cancer."

—Delta Goodrem

One of the first phone calls I received after the press conference came from New York radio and TV personality Ed Randall, host of *Ed Randall's Talking Baseball* on WFAN Sports Radio. Not only is Ed a legendary baseball broadcaster, but he is also a prostate cancer survivor and founder of Ed Randall's Fans for the Cure. He called to encourage me in my cancer battle, and he also wanted to broker a meeting between me and Kathy Giusti, founder of the MMRF. That phone call, in which Ed offered to introduce me to Kathy, was a life changer for me.

Kathy Giusti has done more to advance research and development of drugs and therapies for multiple myeloma than any other person on the planet. I can't thank Ed enough for introducing me to Kathy and the MMRF. Let me take a step back so that Kathy can tell her story in her own words:

I was diagnosed with multiple myeloma in 1996. At the time, I was running worldwide operations for a major pharmaceutical company, G. D. Searle, which is now part of Pfizer. I was thirty-seven, and we had just bought a new home. We had a little girl, eighteen months old. In early December, we were decorating the Christmas tree. I held little Nicole in my arms and smiled at my husband, thinking, *We're so blessed to have such an amazing life.*

A few days later, I had a routine physical, and the tests revealed that I had multiple myeloma. In January, when I packed the Christmas ornaments in the box, I wondered if I'd ever open them again.

At that time, when you were diagnosed with multiple myeloma, you were told you had three years to live—and there was no reason to believe otherwise. There were very few researchers working in the field and very few drugs in the pipeline. This was hard for me to accept as someone working in the pharmaceutical industry.

I called my twin sister, Karen, and said, "You know I'm a very positive person. If there's any hope at all in a situation, I will find it. But, Karen, there's nothing here to hang my hopes on. Nothing."

I might have just pulled the covers over my head—but I had an eighteen-month-old daughter to think of. She saved me. She was so joyful, and when I woke up and looked at her, I just had to smile. I wanted to live long enough that she would remember me. I had heard that if a child knows her mom from the age of five or six, she'll have more memories of her mom. That was my motivation and my goal when my sister, Karen, and I founded the Multiple Myeloma Research Foundation. To date, the Foundation has raised nearly a quarter of a billion dollars for research.

Though Kathy was originally told she had about three years to live, she is in remission today, seventeen years after her diagnosis. One reason: new pharmaceutical advances.

"When the drug Velcade came out," she said, "I was one of the first patients to use it." But the therapy that ultimately saved her life was a stem cell transplant—and the fact that this procedure was even possible at that time was practically a miracle. "I received a stem cell transplant from my identical twin sister," she said. "That was quite a gift from my sister, Karen—and it's rare that a myeloma patient would have an identical twin to serve as a donor."

"I was asleep at the wheel before cancer shook me awake."

—Kris Carr

At the time Kathy was diagnosed, the stem cell transplant procedure I received (called "autologous hematopoietic stem cell transplantation," meaning the harvesting and reimplanting of my own stem cells) was still five years in the future. If Kathy hadn't had a twin sister, she almost certainly would not have survived this long.

Compete Hard—Don't Quit!

While Kathy fought her own cancer battle, she also fought to save many more lives—including, as it turned out, mine.

Kathy brought a whole new strategy to the war against multiple myeloma. Not only has she used her Harvard Business School savvy to raise funds for research, but she has also promoted greater cooperation between pharmaceutical companies and academic centers to invent new drugs. She and her colleagues at the MMRF have created an entirely new clinical network that is enabling research to proceed much faster than ever before.

"We pushed everybody to work together," she says. "The problem we face with an uncommon cancer like myeloma is that one hospital or university medical center may not see enough myeloma patients to amass enough data and tissue for study, or to build a clinical trial. But if you build a network with many centers working together, you create a critical mass of data that enables you to understand how this disease functions and what drugs will work. Clinical networks enable us to move clinical trials faster, and to build tissue banks so we can study myeloma in the laboratory. The result is that in the last ten years, we've seen six new drugs approved by the FDA."

Kathy's efforts have benefited me in a big way. Every time I've run into a problem with one drug, there's always been a new drug for me to try. Those drugs would not exist if not for Kathy Giusti. Kathy and her team get such amazing results by convincing drug companies and university research centers to place their intellectual property—research data that was once a closely guarded secret—into the public domain. When information is shared, it can be studied by the entire research community—and medical advances take place more rapidly.

One of the most promising avenues of research MMRF promotes is genomic sequencing. This technology involves mapping the DNA of cancer cells so that we can better understand what triggers them, what makes one form of cancer different from another, and the best way to destroy cancer cells without harming healthy cells.

Another MMRF innovation is the formation of a large-scale clinical network. Instead of having many small studies conducted by competing research centers on a few dozen patients, researchers network together and pool their data, creating one huge clinical trial involving hundreds or thousands of patients. This creates a wealth of data, which is helping to accelerate the discovery of new treatments and drugs for cancer.

As Kathy shares:

> When I was diagnosed with myeloma, there were three leading centers in the field of myeloma. That was it. Today, there are fifty centers working on our conference trial. When I was diagnosed, hardly any doctors were working in this field. Today, there's an abundance of brilliant, amazing, myeloma doctors.

We've built an inspired community of scientists and clinicians, all sharing data and hypothesizing together, then letting the drug companies see the data so that they can build the right drugs. We are changing the world of cancer research by creating a new open-access world. The result is that we are going to find cancer cures exponentially faster than ever before.

"We are changing the world of cancer research by creating a new open-access world. The result is that we are going to find cancer cures exponentially faster than ever before."

—Kathy Giusti

When we founded MMRF, my goal was to live long enough so that my daughter would remember me. She's nineteen now—and I also have a sixteen-year-old son. I've seen a lot of Christmases since the December when I was diagnosed, and I plan to see many more. It's an amazing gift to turn around and say to myself, *I can't believe I'm still here.* It's been an incredible journey, and I haven't taken one moment of this journey for granted, because every single moment has been a gift.

And I want to say something about the attitude it takes to beat cancer. You couldn't pick a better role model to follow than Pat Williams. There is no quit in this man. I love his passion for living. I love the way he chose a theme for his battle—THE MISSION IS REMISSION. His mission from the beginning was to get his numbers down to zero—complete remission.

Over the years, I've met many cancer patients in person and I've talked to many on the phone. I can tell a lot about people from listening to the sound of their voices. One person will be a dynamo like Pat. The next may sound down and out, completely defeated. You can hear it in their voices—they've given up. Despite my best efforts to find those people the best treatment centers, the best doctors, the best drugs, I'm not at all sure they'll make it. I'm not sure they have the fight in them.

But Pat is all fight. He's the kind of patient every doctor wants to treat, the kind who sees cancer as an opponent to be beaten, the kind who is determined to fight this battle with every ounce of strength he has.

What's fascinating about Pat is that he has been through the gamut. He has been on so many drugs and has not had many windows where he was treatment-free. Compare Pat's treatment to mine—I did several drugs, I had the stem cell transplant, and I've been in a long window where I've been in remission. Pat hasn't had that luxury. It's been an ongoing battle for him.

But Pat never, ever gives up. The last time I talked to him, he said, "My numbers are getting down, Kathy, and I'm going to get them down to zero." He's not going to give up. He's a complete competitor. He's determined to compete hard and to win.

"Cancer affects everyone, and it's up to all of us to support the important research that can one day make a much sought-after cure a reality."

—Angie Harmon

Another character quality every cancer patient needs is a lack of self-pity. People can learn that by watching Pat Williams go through this cancer battle. When you talk to him, there isn't one ounce of feeling sorry for himself. Not ever. Every time I get on the phone with him, I'm struck by the fact that his mission in life is to motivate and inspire others. He's a cheerleader for the patients.

When I met Pat, I thought I would need to cheer him on, but Pat has always been my cheerleader instead. So if you want to be victorious in your cancer battle, learn from Pat Williams. Fight like Pat Williams. Don't feel sorry for yourself—cheer others on like Pat does.

It's incredible what he's done, raising nineteen children (fourteen by international adoption, four by birth, and one by remarriage), winning an NBA championship in Philadelphia, then building a brand-new NBA team from scratch in Orlando. And he's still doing incredible things in his cancer battle today. The same spirit he brought to these other challenges in his life, he now brings to his cancer battle.

If you want to know how to wage a cancer battle, see how Pat does it. Then fight the way he does. Compete hard. Don't give up. Don't quit.

Thanks, Kathy.

To be candid, a part of me feels embarrassed to include Kathy's kind words in this book. But if it helps other people to see how I'm fighting this battle, if my battle can in any way encourage others in their cancer fight, then I'm all for it.

Here's What You Can Do

Dr. Reynolds predicted that the support of the community would be a big factor in my healing—and he was right. If you have given time to serve others in your neighborhood, if you have been a volunteer for community causes, if you have been a tutor to children, if you have been a voice for the voiceless and a defender of the defenseless, your community will remember, and you will be rewarded.

When you have needs, your neighbors will be there for you. When you are hurting, your community will surround you with comfort. When you are in trouble, the people around you will pray for you and reach out to you. And if you are battling cancer, your community will be a resource for healing and recovery.

You may say, "But Pat, I have never engaged in the kind of acts you talk about. I haven't really invested in my community in the past. Is it too late for me to become involved in my community so that my community can become involved in my life?" No! It's not too late! There is so much that you can do even now. Let me give you some suggestions:

1. *Take part in "cancer surveillance" programs.* There are many cancer surveillance programs being conducted all around the world. Cancer surveillance involves the collection and analysis of information on new cancer cases, so that physicians and researchers can better understand the causes of various forms of cancer and how to treat them. The more we know about cancer, the sooner we can cure it.

    Don't worry about an invasion of your privacy. The law requires that any personal, identifying information be removed before the data about your cancer can be transmitted to a cancer database. The only information that is sent is what is known as "de-identified data." Your identity and personal information will always be protected.

By volunteering to participate in cancer surveillance programs, you can turn your adversity into an advantage for finding the cure. There's no single cancer surveillance program that collects data on every form of cancer. There are different programs for myeloma, leukemia, breast cancer, lung cancer, and so on. Ask your doctor how you can participate in a cancer registry, so that information about your cancer can be put to effective use.

"In the future we'll still have cancer,
but we'll detect it very, very early, so that
it won't kill anybody. We'll zap it at
the molecular level decades before
it grows into a tumor."

—Michio Kaku

Examples of major cancer databases include the National Cancer Data Base (NCDB), a joint program of the Commission on Cancer and the American Cancer Society; the National Cancer Institute (NCI) Surveillance, Epidemiology and

End Results (SEER) program; and the National
Program of Cancer Registries (NPCR) of the
Centers for Disease Control and Prevention
(CDC). Ask your oncologist about having your data
shared with the appropriate cancer database.

2. *Take part in clinical trials and studies.* There are many
   different kinds of cancer studies being conducted
   all the time, involving every form of cancer—
   epidemiology studies (which involve the observation
   of participants), prevention studies, screening and
   diagnostic studies, and genomic and biomarker
   studies (providing information about cancer cells at
   the genetic level). Your cancer doctor will be aware
   of studies or trials that you would qualify for.

   A clinical trial is a test of a new cancer
   treatment, such as a cancer drug. If you take part in
   a clinical trial, a doctor or researcher will explain to
   you the reason for the study and the risks involved.
   After signing a consent form, you'll receive the best
   currently accepted treatment for your cancer, or a
   new treatment that doctors hope will be even better
   than the standard treatment. By studying how you
   respond to treatment during the trial, doctors will
   learn how to better treat your form of cancer in the
   future. Those who participate in clinical trials are
   usually the first to receive cutting-edge treatments.

If you have been diagnosed with multiple myeloma, consider participating in clinical studies such as the MMRF CoMMpass study, which collects tissue samples and analyzes genetic information from myeloma patients. Learn more about this and other myeloma-related clinical studies at http://www.themmrf.org/.

3. *Help spread the word about cancer.* In conversations with friends and neighbors, and in discussions at social media sites, help spread the facts about cancer. Let people know that it's okay to talk about cancer. Tell your friends that cancer is not an automatic death sentence but a disease that can usually be managed, controlled, and frequently cured. Spread the word that nearly two-thirds of people diagnosed with cancer are still alive five years after their initial diagnosis—and the survival rate is improving all the time. According to the American Association for Cancer Research, there are now almost 14 million cancer survivors in the United States today, with a million being added each year.[11] And let

> Let people know that it's okay to talk about cancer. Tell your friends that cancer is not an automatic death sentence but a disease that can usually be managed, controlled, and frequently cured.

your friends know that one-third of cancers can be prevented if we make the right choices about diet, exercise, smoking, and environmental pollutants.

Friends and family members of cancer patients can set up cancer tribute pages to talk about your treatment experiences and to enable others to offer messages of encouragement and support. Or you can set up your own blog or online journal to talk about your cancer journey.

4. *Get involved in consciousness-raising and fund-raising events.* Many cancer organizations, such as the MMRF, hold events to raise cancer awareness and raise funds for cancer research. At these events, you will meet other patients and family members who share your experience. By making connections with others who have been touched by cancer, you'll find strength in numbers. You may want to join with the people you meet to start a support group or a fund-raising effort in your community. Examples of fund-raising events include 5K walk/runs, marathons or half-marathons, cycling events, or charity golf tournaments. Contact a reputable organization or foundation (such as the MMRF) for information and assistance in starting such events in your community.

5. *Donate.* There are many meaningful ways to donate to cancer research. Examples: Donate in honor or memory of a loved one. Donate through planned giving (that is, making a bequest in your will). Donate a vehicle. Give a recurring gift on a monthly or annual basis. If you are a business owner, offer to match donations made by your employees or customers (an excellent way to motivate others to give generously).

6. *Start or join a cancer support group.* I have spoken to the multiple myeloma support group in Orlando—a group of about thirty people who are at different stages in their myeloma battle. They have a potluck supper and talk about their triumphs, struggles, and experiences with myeloma. Every city needs a cancer support group, and probably a support group for every kind of cancer. If there's no support group in your city, consider starting one. The need is great—and the moment you announce it, you'll be amazed at the response.

Cancer Is Not the Worst Thing

Pastor James is intensely involved in the community, and in the battle against cancer. He shares:

I've been asked to speak many times at American Cancer Society events, as well as to churches and organizations. I'm quick to point out that a person who has cancer is not the only one affected by cancer. Spouses, family members, and close friends of cancer patients are also affected. In fact, cancer impacts the entire community, not only because of its financial costs, but because it so often robs us of the priceless contributions of the people around us.

Cancer is something we wouldn't wish on our worst enemies. Medical science has made great strides in developing cancer drugs and chemotherapies that are less harsh than some of the old approaches. Years ago, I underwent chemo that was so horrible, I don't know how I could have gotten through it without God's strength.

"I attacked my cancer diagnosis
the same way I attack training
and competing, and that's
pretty fearless."

—Eric Shanteau

But even with all I've gone through with cancer, I have to say that cancer is not the worst thing in the world. There is a famous poem by Robert L. Lynn called "Cancer Is So

Limited." Lynn lists all the things that cancer cannot steal from us—love, hope, peace, friendship, faith, courage, and memories. Above all, cancer cannot take away our eternal life, if we have faith in Jesus Christ. Cancer is not the worst thing in the world.

What's worse than cancer? Living in isolation from friends and family. Living without any connection to our community. Living and dying without faith in Jesus Christ.

I truly believe that medical science will find a cure for cancer—maybe in our lifetime. Researchers are learning how cancer works at the DNA level, and this new and deeper understanding of cancer is producing new approaches all the time. Whenever I talk to people who are battling cancer, I say, "Don't ever, ever give up! They could find a cure tomorrow."

And that's no empty cliché. The hope of an ultimate cure for cancer is the second-greatest hope in the world, second only to the hope of eternal life through Christ. I absolutely believe the cure for cancer is just around the corner.

Pastor Randall James is right: Medical science is advancing, and cancer is retreating—but cancer is taking as many casualties as it can along the way. We mustn't let up. We have to keep fighting until the war on cancer is won, once and for all.

EPILOGUE:
THE PRIVILEGE OF CANCER

As I write these words, I'm in the fourth year of my cancer battle.

On the day Dr. Reynolds first told me I had cancer, he also said, "Our mission is to keep you alive long enough for all these new treatments to come into the pipeline."

And sure enough, every year there's been another drug, another therapy, another weapon in the battle against multiple myeloma. The next three years of my cancer battle have already been mapped out. I know exactly what's coming, year by year by year. I'm currently on a drug that was just approved in the last six months. I started that drug in the spring of 2013. The good news is that it's a pill, so I can swallow this chemo with a glass of water instead of spending two four-hour sessions in the chemo chair on successive days.

The new treatments and medications that Dr. Reynolds promised are coming into the pipeline, just as he said. So the fight goes on.

If there's one thing I've learned in this battle, it's that cancer is going to do whatever it's going to do. You can't reason with cancer. You can't bargain with cancer. You can't scare cancer off with threats.

When cancer attacks, you have a choice to make: fight or surrender. Once you make the choice to fight, you realize you have many weapons at your disposal. You have the latest medical technology, the latest therapies and drugs, and the most committed doctors and nurses you'll ever meet.

You also discover that you have some weapons at your disposal that you never knew you had. One of the most potent of these weapons is the ability to choose your attitude. I could have chosen to sit in my backyard and watch life go by, waiting to die. But I decided to make a different choice. I decided to fight hard. I decided to remain optimistic and hopeful. I decided to stay engaged in my life and career. I decided to plan for the future, and to take the steps to ensure that I would be around in the future to see my plans come true.

Cancer doesn't own me. Cancer hasn't defeated me. Cancer doesn't call the shots. I don't have time to sit around and worry about cancer. I'm too busy living my life, enjoying my family, and getting things done.

A journalist recently asked me, "Pat, if you had a chance to rewind your life and relive these past few years without cancer, would you do it?" When he asked me that question, he was interviewing me during a chemo session, while a cancer drug was dripping into the port in my chest.

> Cancer doesn't own me.
> Cancer hasn't defeated me.
> Cancer doesn't call the shots.
> I don't have time to sit around and worry about cancer.
> I'm too busy living my life, enjoying my family, and getting things done.

My reflex answer would have been, "Of course! Look at what I'm doing right now! I'm going through a chemo session as we speak! Who wouldn't want to have a normal life instead of being hooked up to all these tubes and machines?"

But after just a few seconds of reflection, I realized that the answer off the top of my head was not the true answer. I said, "Would I trade these past few years for the chance to have my normal life back? Honestly, I don't think I would."

The reporter looked at me with surprise plainly written on his face—and probably a touch of disbelief.

"I'm no masochist," I said. "I certainly don't enjoy all I've gone through with this cancer. But I honestly consider it a privilege to be tested this way."

"A privilege . . . to have cancer?"

"Look at it this way: We all want to leave an imprint on the next generation, don't we? We want our lives to count for something. We want to make a difference. We want to make an impact on others. We want to be able to look back on our lives and say, 'My life mattered. God used my life to influence others.' Yes, the things I've done in the sports world mattered, my books and speeches mattered, my children and grandchildren *really* mattered. But when it's all said and done, I think the way I've fought this cancer battle may be the most significant thing I have ever done with my life."

"How is that?"

"I've been able to help promote research and help fund the construction of a multiple myeloma center at Florida Hospital. I've been a laboratory rat for a lot of new medical technologies that may eventually lead to a cure. Through my media exposure during my cancer battle, I've been able to give people hope and encouragement. I've tried to serve as a role model of optimism and perseverance for others who are going through their own cancer battle. I could never have done all of that if I hadn't had the privilege of having multiple myeloma, could I?"

I have to be honest: I haven't always viewed cancer as a privilege. When I first learned that I had been diagnosed with an incurable cancer, I was pretty shaken up. I couldn't understand at first why God would allow this to happen in my life.

But I thank God that he didn't allow me to wallow in self-pity. I remember saying to Dr. Reynolds during that visit,

"This is hard, but I'll be all right. For seventy-plus years, I've lived quite a charmed life. I've had so many amazing experiences, met so many incredible people, and been an eyewitness to so many events. Not many people get the opportunities I've had. So, Doc, if my life has to end soon, I have to say it's been a very full life. I want to keep living to see my grandchildren grow up, and I'm going to fight this cancer with everything I've got—but if I have to go, I'm ready. I'm not afraid to die."

"Having had cancer,
one important thing to know
is you're still the same person at the end.
You're stripped down to near zero.
But most people come out the other end
feeling more like themselves
than ever before."

—Kylie Minogue

I still feel that way. I'm optimistic, I'm fighting the good fight, I'm competing hard against cancer—yet I'm not afraid to die.

I'm not going to wait around to die. I'm going to live my life and keep reaching for my goals and dreams. I'm going to keep scheduling my priorities and making plans for the future. Cancer or no cancer, I expect to be here for a good long while.

I'll admit, I haven't always been the perfect patient. I haven't always gotten the bed rest my doctors recommended. When my immune system was compromised, I didn't always keep myself isolated from other people as my doctors would have wished. It's not that I'm stubborn or that I don't care about my health. It's that I'm still focused on my goals and objectives, and living my life. I know I have cancer, but I'm not focused on cancer.

I have always tried to be an obedient patient, to do as my doctor recommends. But there have been times when I've had to weigh doctor's orders against the prospect of being imprisoned by this disease. Occasionally, I overdo it. But overall, I've found a pretty good balance.

I remember the 2012 NBA All-Star Weekend. It took place in Orlando in late February, and I had just undergone my stem cell transplant. Hosting the event was a big honor for the Orlando Magic, and I didn't want to miss any of it. Though my doctors had predicted I would be in the hospital for three weeks, I was out in a record-setting ten days. I could no more spend the All-Star Weekend in a hospital room than a seven-year-old could spend Christmas morning in his bedroom.

I planned to be careful and to limit my contact with other people as much as possible, since I essentially had no immune system. I was supposed to be in isolation, and if I went out, I was supposed to wear a surgical mask. Well, I got out of the hospital on Tuesday, and I had a speaking event on Wednesday, two on Thursday, one event on Saturday morning, another on Saturday night, a Sunday morning chapel, plus, I was guest of honor and featured speaker at an NBA Legends brunch later on Sunday.

Did my doctors know my itinerary for the All-Star Weekend? No way! And I wasn't going to tell them. Dr. Reynolds is soft-spoken and mild-mannered—I could endure his gentle scolding. But I was afraid of Dr. Khaled! I was sure that if he knew where I was going and what I was doing that weekend, he'd have me skinned alive. I knew he wouldn't want me out among the crowds, risking his perfect record of successful transplants.

Though I made a number of public appearances and faced many crowds, I never wore a surgical mask. But I was careful to minimize my exposure to disease-causing microbes. I have learned that if you want to stay well, you have to wash your hands frequently with soap and warm water, then grab a clean paper towel to avoid contact with door handles and other surfaces. When people reached toward me for a handshake, I'd turn it into a fist bump and say, "Germ free!" And I carried alcohol-based hand sanitizer with me wherever I went.

One thing I didn't count on while I was going to various activities at the NBA All-Star Weekend was that my NBA

Legends speech would be broadcast on the NBA TV chan-
nel—and that Dr. Khaled, my Knicks-fan stem cell transplant
doctor, would be watching live from his living room! I had
tried so hard to keep him from finding out what I was doing
that weekend—but I had no control over the TV cameras.
So there I was, as big as life on Dr. Khaled's flat-screen TV,
wearing my Indiana Jones hat, disobeying his orders, giving
a speech instead of isolating myself from the big, bad, germy
world. The next time I was in Dr. Khaled's office, I heard
about it. Oh, boy, did I hear about it!

So my advice to you is to face your cancer squarely, follow doctor's orders as much as possible, wash your hands
frequently, and follow every possible precaution against
germs—but don't live as an invalid
or a victim. Get on with your life!
Focus on your goals! Live passion-
ately and joyfully and optimisti-
cally! Don't make cancer the focus
of your life. Make *life* the focus of
your life!

Throughout this book I have
been talking to three audiences:
(1) people who have been diagnosed with cancer, (2) people
who are helping and encouraging loved ones in their cancer battles, and (3) people who are healthy now but who
know that cancer may play a role in their lives someday. My

six-point message throughout this book is that no matter where you are in your cancer journey, it's not too late to start building six all-important resources into your life:

1. **A Positive Outlook**
2. **Keeping Fit**
3. **A Durable Faith**
4. **A Loving Family**
5. **Caring Friends**
6. **A Supportive Community**

These six resources can make all the difference in your cancer battle. Whether you are a cancer patient, the loved one of a cancer patient, or someone who is preparing for a potential cancer battle in the future, your mission is remission. Your mission may be your own remission, the remission of someone you love, or even the remission of people you've never met. We are at war with cancer, and we are fighting our battles with weapons of prayer, optimism, activism, fundraising, and awareness-raising efforts.

"As a cancer doctor, I'm looking forward to being out of a job."

—Daniel Kraft, M.D.

During one of my visits to Florida Hospital for treatment, I was looking at a bulletin board in the hall, and I noticed a poem called "Fight for Life," which Lorna Mahan had written for her teenage son Sinjin, who has been battling Burkitt's lymphoma since 2007. She wrote:

> *Storms of life are strong enough*
> *without cancer stepping in,*
> *Came creeping through the back door*
> *just counting on a win.*
> *Engaging you in battle*
> *we firmly stand our ground,*
> *Armed with courage, faith and hope,*
> *our child's life we surround.*
> *This fight rages day and night*
> *the will to survive is strong,*
> *We will never surrender*
> *In our lives you don't belong.*
> *Prepare yourself to lose this time*
> *our child's life you won't take,*
> *This is a fight you will not win*
> *Cancer, make no mistake!*[12]

Lorna Mahan expresses the prayer of my heart, and I'm sure the prayer of your heart as well. Wherever you are in your journey, I pray you will become a warrior in the battle against cancer. Fight hard. Begin each day with optimism and end each day with hope for tomorrow. Persevere. Never give up.

The day is coming, and I believe it's coming soon, when we will be able to say, "Mission accomplished! Cancer has been vanquished!"

Until that day comes, we fight on. And we fight to win.

NOTES

1 National Cancer Institute, "Lifetime Risk of Developing or Dying from Cancer," Cancer.org, November 29, 2012, http://www.cancer.org/cancer/cancerbasics/lifetime-probability-of-developing-or-dying-from-cancer.

2 National Cancer Institute, "Cancer of All Sites—SEER Stat Fact Sheets," US Department of Health and Human Services, National Institutes of Health, National Cancer Institute, November 2012, http://seer.cancer.gov/statfacts/html/all.html#survival.

3 Lucia Giuggio Carvalho, RN, MSN, and James A. Stewart, MD, "Develop a Positive Mental Attitude," NetPlaces.com, Living with Breast Cancer, 2009, http://www.netplaces.com/living-with-breast-cancer/positive-mental-attitude/develop-a-positive-mental-attitude.htm.

4 Science News, "Lung Cancer Patients with Optimistic Attitudes Have Longer Survival, Study Finds," International Association for the Study of Lung Cancer (March 8, 2010), *ScienceDaily*, http://www.sciencedaily.com/releases/2010/03/100303131656.htm.

5 Rich DeVos, *Hope from My Heart: 10 Lessons for Life* (Nashville, TN: Thomas Nelson, 2000), 44.

6 Ryan Tate, "Harvard Cancer Expert: Steve Jobs Probably Doomed Himself with Alternative Medicine," Gawker.com, October 13, 2011, http://gawker.com/5849543/harvard-cancer-expert-steve-jobs-probably-doomed-himself-with-alternative-medicine.

7 John Piper, *A Sweet and Bitter Providence: Sex, Race, and the Sovereignty of God* (Wheaton, IL: Crossway, 2010), 101–2.

8 Randolph C. Byrd, MD, "Positive Therapeutic Effects of Intercessory Prayer in a Coronary Care Unit Population," *Southern Medical Journal* 81, no. 7 (July 1988): 829.

9 Eric Adler, Knight Ridder, Athens Newspapers, Inc., "Heart Patients May Benefit from Other People's Prayers," http://onlineathens.com/stories/102799/hea_1027990042.shtml.

10 "Rest in the Hope," words & music by Karyn Williams / Brian White / Trey Heffinger. Copyright © 2012 Meaux Jeaux Music / Tunes From the Basement / Admin: EMICMGPublishing.com/SESAC/Songs From Cincy/SESAC/Only Youtunes/SESAC. Available on iTunes. Artist's website at www.karynwilliams.com. Used by permission.

11 Kelly Fitzgerald, "By 2022 There Will Be Nearly 18 Million Cancer Survivors in the US," MedicalNewsToday.com, March 28, 2013, http://www.medicalnewstoday.com/articles/258320.php.

12 Lorna Mahan, "Fight for Life," FamilyFriendPoems.com, http://www.familyfriendpoems.com/poem/fight-for-life.

AUTHOR INFORMATION

You can contact Pat Williams at:

Pat Williams
c/o Orlando Magic
8701 Maitland Summit Boulevard
Orlando, FL 32810
phone: 407-916-2404
pwilliams@orlandomagic.com

Visit Pat Williams's website at:

www.PatWilliams.com
On Twitter: @OrlandoMagicPat

If you would like to set up a speaking engagement with Pat Williams, please call or write his assistant, Andrew Herdliska, at the above address or call him at 407-916-2401. Requests can also be faxed to 407-916-2986 or e-mailed to aherdliska@orlandomagic.com.

We would love to hear from you. Please send your comments about this book to Pat Williams. Thank you.

PAT WILLIAMS

Founder and Vice President, The Orlando Magic

Dear Friend,

I hope this book has encouraged and strengthened you. I've been encouraged to look back over these events and see how God has led me through my cancer battle. I believe God calls us at key moments in our lives to face a challenge, to serve Him, to serve others, and to discover deeper levels of character and faith within us. He rarely calls us at a time that's convenient for us—but when He calls, we must answer.

When I first learned of my diagnosis with multiple myeloma and began my treatments, a longtime friend asked me if I was going to write a book about my experience. At the time, I was too focused on my treatments and the emotions of facing multiple myeloma to think about writing a book.

Yet, God called me again. I sensed Him telling me it was time to write this book. During the past three years, I've learned a great deal about cancer, and especially multiple myeloma. For example, I was surprised to learn that there was no comprehensive multiple myeloma center in the southeastern United States, and that few centers exist in the United States. I discovered that a patient is *five times more likely to survive* multiple myeloma when treated at a comprehensive center. I love those odds— and I wondered how we might bring such a facility to central Florida.

During my course of treatment, I was continually amazed by the talent, dedication, compassion, and skill of the doctors and nurses at Florida Hospital in Orlando, I realized that these professionals would be the perfect foundation for a regional multiple myeloma center. I sensed that God was calling me once again—this time to help build a comprehensive multiple myeloma center in Orlando.

I'm passionate about this project. I'm committed to seeing a major regional Multiple Myeloma Center right here at Florida Hospital. I'm committed to doing everything I can to make this dream a reality.

Years ago I was part of a magnificent team of people who defied the odds and brought an NBA franchise—the Orlando Magic—to central Florida. It was a lot of work, but now I know what it takes to beat the odds. It takes a dedicated team of like-minded people.

Every person who battles cancer and accomplishes the mission of remission is an odds-beater, a champion, a warrior against this disease. With your help I hope we can do it again by developing a center of excellence in Orlando that will care for patients throughout the region and across the country.

Won't you consider joining me in this incredible effort? To become part of the team that makes Magic happen one more time, please visit www.magiconemoretime.com and make a gift today.

Thank you and God bless you,
Pat